METHADONE MAINTENANCE TREATMENT IN THE U.S.

ABOUT THE AUTHORS

DR. WENDEE WECHSBERG is the director of the Substance Abuse Treatment Evaluations and Interventions Research Program at RTI International. Dr. Wechsberg has more than two decades of clinical experience and she has directed outpatient drug-free, methadone, and residential substance abuse treatment programs. She is currently conducting intervention research in the United States and South Africa to help women who abuse substances to reduce violence and victimization, and to decrease the spread of HIV. She has published in the areas of methadone treatment, outreach, HIV risk behaviors, and gender and intervention effectiveness.

DR. JENNIFER KASTEN is a senior health policy analyst in the Substance Abuse Treatment Evaluations and Interventions Research Program at RTI International. Dr. Kasten has conducted extensive substance abuse treatment research and she is an experienced substance abuse treatment counselor. Currently, she is examining the impact of institutional and market forces on organizational change through federal regulations, and she is working on a SAMHSA project to facilitate data collection and analysis of national outcome measures by states for substance abuse treatment. Dr. Kasten received her doctorate in Public Administration in December 2006.

DR. NANCY BERKMAN is a research analyst in the Health Care Organization, Delivery, and Access Program at RTI International. Dr. Berkman specializes in health policy and health services research studies, including delivery of substance abuse treatment, particularly racial/ethnic disparities in access to support services and methadone treatment outcomes. She is also currently studying patterns of care received by insured women with ovarian cancer and cervical cytological abnormalities. She has led systematic evidence-based reviews of the literature concerning management of preterm labor, literacy and health outcomes, and the management of eating disorders.

DR. AMY ROUSSEL is an organizational sociologist in the Health Care Organization, Delivery, and Access Program at RTI International. Dr. Roussel specializes in public health services research. Her expertise includes both qualitative and quantitative research in the areas of public health systems, health services, health policy and management, substance abuse treatment, performance measurement, and program evaluation. In addition, she has led and contributed to a variety of multidisciplinary teams, encompassing tasks such as primary data collection, case study analysis, analysis of secondary data, and policy analysis.

METHADONE MAINTENANCE TREATMENT IN THE U.S.

A PRACTICAL QUESTION AND ANSWER GUIDE

Wendee M. Wechsberg & Jennifer J. Kasten

with contributions from Nancy D. Berkman & Amy E. Roussel

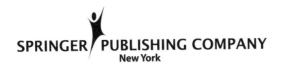

SPRINGER PUBLISHING COMPANY
New York

Springer Publishing Company, LLC
11 West 42nd Street
New York, NY 10036
www.springerpub.com

Acquisitions Editor: Jennifer Perillo
Production Editor: Rose Mary Piscitelli
Cover design: Shari Lambert and John Theilgard
Composition: International Graphic Services

07 08 09 10 / 5 4 3 2 1

Library of Congress Cataloging-in-Publication Data

Wechsberg, Wendee M.
    Methadone maintenance treatment in the U.S. : a practical question and answer guide / Wendee M. Wechsberg & Jennifer J. Kasten with contributions from Nancy D. Berkman & Amy E. Roussel.
        p. ; cm.
    Includes bibliographical references and index.
    ISBN 978-0-8261-0130-3 (alk. paper)
    1. Methadone maintenance--United States--Miscellanea. I. Kasten, Jennifer J. II. Title.
    [DNLM: 1. Methadone--therapeutic use--United States. 2. Opioid-Related Disorders--rehabilitation--United States. 3. Substance Abuse Treatment Centers--organization & administration--United States. WM 284 W386m 2007]

RC568.M4W43 2007
362.196'8632061--dc22

                                                                    2007006240

Printed in the United States of America by Bang Printing

ABOUT RTI INTERNATIONAL

RTI International is dedicated to conducting research and development that improves the human condition by turning knowledge into practice. With a staff of more than 2,500, RTI offers innovative research and technical solutions to governments and businesses worldwide in the areas of health and pharmaceuticals, education and training, surveys and statistics, democratic governance, economic and social development, advanced technology, energy, and the environment.

The second largest independent nonprofit research organization in the United States, RTI maintains nine offices in the U.S., five international offices, and one international subsidiary, as well as project offices around the world.

DEDICATION

This book is dedicated to Dr. Herman Diesenhaus, who departed this life too soon and before the completion of this work to which he contributed so significantly. Dr. Diesenhaus was not only the government project officer who brought this project to life and to closure, he was also the force and the will behind this endeavor. He challenged us at every turn and guided us toward completion. We honor his unwavering spirit by sharing this book. Dr. Diesenhaus had been a program director and a state methadone authority, and he was a giant in his commitment to the field of methadone maintenance treatment. His thoughts and beliefs permeate this book, and he will be with us always in heart and spirit.

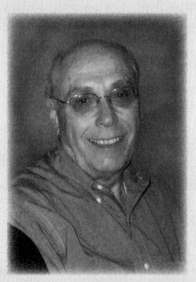

In Memoriam
October 1, 1938 – May 16, 2006

CONTENTS

PREFACE

To date, there has been no comprehensive, user-friendly professional reference book based on information from a large sample of methadone maintenance treatment (MMT) programs in the United States. This book fills this gap. It is written for a diverse audience, including clinicians, program administrators, policy makers, substance abuse treatment researchers, and other health service professionals who want to learn about all aspects of MMT. We hope to offer insights into the new regulatory standards for MMT, as well as an overview of MMT in the United States today. We also hope that policy makers interested in establishing new MMT programs, domestically and internationally, will find the information useful—particularly because of the demonstrated relationship between heroin use and the spread of AIDS, which necessitates exploring and expanding proven harm-reduction strategies.

There are more than 1,200 MMT programs in the United States, with an estimated staff of over 20,000. Despite the magnitude of these programs, frontline staff have limited professional resources that are both user-friendly and empirically based. Lessons garnered from the past 40 years of MMT can provide guidance on numerous dimensions of program implementation and service delivery, including program practices and personnel, policies and regulation, effective screening and assessment tools, access to services, patient characteristics, specialized care, quality assurance and patient satisfaction, cost of services, and the impact of accreditation on MMT.

We hope that this book, which is drawn from the Evaluation of the Opioid Treatment Accreditation Study (Center for Substance Abuse Treatment, Contract No. 270-97-7002), will help bring the domains of MMT research and practice closer together. The distilled findings presented here offer practical guidance on compliance with the new accreditation standards, as well as additional recommendations for quality assurance procedures. This critical information will enable MMT program administrators and staff to continue building a treatment system that maintains or exceeds required standards of care while improving client access to services that are supportive, comprehensive, and effective.

Wendee Wechsberg
Jennifer Kasten

ACKNOWLEDGMENTS

The original study on which this book is based was supported by the Center for Substance Abuse Treatment (CSAT) under Contract No. 270-97-7002 to RTI International. We gratefully acknowledge the special contribution of Kathleen N. Lohr, who was instrumental in developing the research, and the support of Herman Diesenhaus, the CSAT Project Officer. Additionally, we would like to thank CSAT's Division of Pharmacological Therapies, specifically, Robert Lubran, Ray Hylton, Arlene Stanton, and Nick Reuter. We also would like to acknowledge the work of Bill Luckey and Lori Ducharme, who initiated the original study. We thank Tom D'Aunno, Teresa Goens, Steve Magura, Ira Marion, J. Thomas Payte, Janice Kauffman, and Stephen Molinari, who worked with us as consultants on the project. We would like to thank Rick Harwood and Ansari Ameen for their insights and contributions as subcontractors during the early work of the project. We offer our deep gratitude to the methadone maintenance treatment programs, their staff, and their patients who took the time to share their experiences. Without their participation, this project would not have been possible. We thank Gary Zarkin, who guided the research in his role as lead economist, and Laura Dunlap as senior economist. We are indebted to Sheila Knight, who led the multiyear data collection process necessary to complete this work, and Georgiy Bobashev, who served as lead analyst on the project. We are especially grateful to Larry Crum, Barbara Flannery, and Erika Fulmer, each of whom authored individual chapters for the final CSAT project report. We want to especially thank Will Meyer, Siobhan Young, and Linda Allen for their support of our writing needs. We recognize the invaluable contributions of Jeff Novey, Lauren Mine, Kathleen Mohar, Shari Lambert, and Diane Eckard, whose editorial, production coordination, and graphics skills contributed significantly to the quality of this work. Finally, we would like to sincerely thank Vice President Wayne Holden and President Victoria Haynes of RTI for their support of this book.

LIST OF ACRONYMS AND ABBREVIATIONS

AAL	Accreditation Activity Log
AATOD	American Association for the Treatment of Opioid Dependence
ADSS	Alcohol and Drug Services Study
AMA	American Medical Association
ARV	antiretroviral
ASAM	American Society of Addiction Medicine
ASI	Addiction Severity Index
AUDIT	Alcohol Use Disorders Identification Test
CAC	Certified Addiction Counselor
CADAC	Certified Alcohol and Drug Abuse Counselor
CAGE	Cut Down, Annoyed, Guilty Eye Opener
CALDATA	California Drug And Alcohol Treatment Assessment
CARF	Commission on Accreditation of Rehabilitation Facilities
CDAC	Certified Drug Abuse Counselor
CEWG	Community Epidemiology Work Group
CHAMPUS	Civilian Health and Medical Program of the Uniformed Services
CLIA	Clinical Laboratory Improvement Act of 1988 (CLIA)
CMS	Centers for Medicare and Medicaid Services
COA	Council on Accreditation
CSA	Controlled Substances Act
CSAT	Center for Substance Abuse Treatment
DARP	Drug Abuse Reporting Program
DASIS	Drug and Alcohol Services Information System
DAST	Drug Abuse Screening Test
DATOS	Drug Abuse Treatment Outcome Studies
DAWN	Drug Abuse Warning Network
DEA	Drug Enforcement Agency
DHHS	Department of Health and Human Services
DSM-IV	Diagnostic and Statistical Manual of Mental Disorders, Fourth Edition
FDA	Food and Drug Administration
GAO	Government Accountability Office (formerly General Accounting Office)
HBV	hepatitis B virus

HCV	hepatitis C virus
HIV/AIDS	Human Immunodeficiency Virus/Acquired Immunodeficiency Syndrome
IDU	injecting drug user
INTPRB	Interagency Narcotic Treatment and Policy Review Board
IOM	Institute of Medicine
JCAHO	Joint Commission on Accreditation of Healthcare Organizations
LAAM	levo-alpha-acetyl-methadol
MAST	Michigan Alcoholism Screening Test
MMT	methadone maintenance treatment
MSM	men who have sex with men
MTQAS	Methadone Treatment Quality Assurance System
NATA	Narcotic Addiction Treatment Act of 1974
NEP	needle exchange program
NIDA	National Institute on Drug Abuse
NIH	National Institutes of Health
NIMH	National Institute of Mental Health
NSDUH	National Survey on Drug Use and Health
N-SSATS	National Survey of Substance Abuse Treatment Services
NTIES	National Treatment Improvement Evaluation Study
OAS	Office of Applied Studies
PATS	Partnership Attitude Tracking Study
QA	Quality Assurance
RN	Registered Nurse
SAMHSA	Substance Abuse and Mental Health Services Administration
SAODAP	Special Action Officer of Drug Abuse Policy
SAPT	Substance Abuse Prevention and Treatment
SASSI	Substance Abuse Subtle Screening Inventory
SEP	syringe exchange program
SMA	state methadone authority
SROS	Services Research Outcomes Study
TB	tuberculosis
TEDS	Treatment Episode Data Set
TOPS	Treatment Outcome Prospective Study

CHAPTER 1—Introduction

Although methadone maintenance has been the primary form of treatment for opiate dependence for over 40 years, no previous resource has offered providers and policy makers a broad range of well-supported, practical information in a user-friendly format. This chapter provides an overview of methadone maintenance treatment (MMT), covering the need for this book, the scope and history of opiate dependence and MMT, and the context of dependence and treatment.

WHY DO WE NEED A USER-FRIENDLY BOOK ON METHADONE TREATMENT?

The field of methadone treatment has expanded immensely over the past four decades, yet there have been no large domestic studies on the comprehensive MMT service system since 1991, when Ball and Ross published *The Effectiveness of Methadone Maintenance Treatment: Patients, Programs, Services, and Outcomes.* Further, the existing publications, though capturing dimensions of MMT, are not in a format immediately useful to clinicians, policy makers, and researchers.

The need for a user-friendly book is clear, especially as the abuse of heroin and other opiates continues to be a serious public health problem. Opiate dependence is increasing worldwide and significantly exacerbating the HIV/AIDS pandemic (Cooper, 1989; Metzger et al., 1993). In the United States, most opiate dependence therapy is in the form of MMT, which serves more than 200,000 patients annually. MMT has been shown to help opiate abusers stabilize their lives, allowing them to become productive employees and fully functioning members of their family and community (Dole, 1988; Dole & Nyswander, 1965; Phillips et al., 1995).

Although MMT is a widely used and accepted treatment modality, it is not uncontroversial. As a drug replacement therapy intended to reduce harm, MMT can last for many years, particularly in programs that focus on minimizing opiate use and its negative consequences rather than on complete abstinence. Without treatment, however, many opiate abusers would continue a drug-using lifestyle and would therefore be at increased risk of criminal involvement and infectious diseases.

Opiate dependence attracted heightened media attention during the mid- to late-1990s, when heroin-related emergency department episodes tripled in the United States (U.S. Department of Health and Human Services [DHHS], 2001b). In response to the growing AIDS crisis, which was attributable in part to an increase in injecting drug use, almost every MMT program in the United States significantly increased its capacity, helping stabilize injecting use–related AIDS cases over the past decade.

Unfortunately, injecting drug use, especially heroin use, continues to increase globally, as does the associated risk of disease. The risk is particularly high in Western European and Eurasian countries. For example, injecting drug use accounts for 65% of AIDS cases in Spain and 91% of cases in Kazakhstan (Aceijas, Stimson, Hickman, & Rhodes, 2004). Many foreign governments are only starting to consider MMT programs as a treatment response and need to learn more about how it functions in the United States.

This book is a primer on MMT, including how programs are structured and staffed, and the components of service delivery. We hope that its format clearly presents the data we collected during a national methadone study, encouraging broader treatment for opiate dependence.

WHAT IS METHADONE MAINTENANCE TREATMENT?

In a clinical setting, substituting a less addictive opiate (e.g., methadone) for a more addictive one (e.g., heroin) and then tapering and maintaining the dosage of the substitution opiate over time is now a well-established technique for reducing illicit opiate use. Legally, methadone can be provided only in strictly regulated, clinically observed environments that limit take-home doses. As a result, patients are required to present regularly to federally approved MMT programs for assessment and medication prescription. For new patients, this means daily visits to an MMT program to receive a dose of medication from medical staff. MMT, which often has long waiting lists, is restricted to individuals with documented histories of chronic opiate dependence. Individuals who have only recently developed opiate dependence are ineligible.

The search for safe, office-based alternative treatments for opiate dependence may yield new ways to reach more individuals. Taken orally, methadone is stored in the liver and is metabolized more slowly than injected opiates. One proposed office-based treatment is a tablet formulation of buprenorphine (a semisynthetic opioid whose pain-relieving effect lasts longer than that of morphine) and naloxone (which can diminish the potential for buprenorphine abuse).

MMT is a highly regulated pharmacologic adjunctive treatment for opiate dependence. Over 1,200 MMT programs are approved to operate in the United States. These programs vary in types of services offered, staff backgrounds and credentials, capacity, dosing practices, and caseloads.

WHAT ARE SOME PHARMACOLOGIC ALTERNATIVES TO METHADONE TREATMENT?

Buprenorphine. Buprenorphine is a partial opioid (synthetic opiate) agonist. Although it is an opiate and thus can produce typical opiate agonist effects and side effects, such as euphoria and respiratory depression, buprenorphine's maximal effects are less than those of full agonists, such as heroin and methadone. At low doses, buprenorphine produces sufficient agonist effects to enable opiate-dependent individuals to discontinue abuse without experiencing withdrawal symptoms. The agonist effects of buprenorphine increase linearly with increasing doses but plateau at moderate doses. This is known as the ceiling effect. Thus, compared with full agonists, buprenorphine carries a lower risk of abuse, dependence, and side effects. In high doses, buprenorphine can, in fact, block the effects of full agonists and can precipitate withdrawal symptoms if administered to opiate-dependent individuals who have a full agonist in their bloodstream.

Formulations for opiate dependence treatment are sublingual tablets. Because of the ceiling effect and poor bioavailability, buprenorphine is safer in overdose than full agonists. The maximal effects of buprenorphine appear to occur in the 16- to 32-mg dose range for sublingual tablets. Higher doses are unlikely to produce greater effects.

Buprenorphine can be used successfully for low-dose opiate abusers, who can be medically monitored on a less frequent basis. This medication has also been found to be helpful with HIV infection because of its adherence to antiretroviral (ARV) medications. There is a ceiling effect, however, for patients with a high tolerance to opiates. A significant barrier to greater utilization of buprenorphine in MMT programs in the United States is the cost of the drug and the lack of insurance coverage.

Naloxone. Naloxone is a drug used to reverse the effects of opium and its derivatives (heroin, morphine, and codeine). It can be used as a life-saving measure in narcotic overdose situations by countering depression of the central nervous and respiratory systems. The drug has been shown to reduce rates of fatal overdoses when included as part of emergency kits for heroin users. It can also be given to newborn infants whose mothers have received opium-like drugs. For quickest action, naloxone is usually injected. It begins to act in about 2 minutes, and its effects typically last 45 minutes. It is marketed under the trade names Narcan, Nalone, and Narcanti.

Naltrexone. Naltrexone is an opioid receptor antagonist used for rapid opiate detoxification, which decreases patients' withdrawal symptoms by producing an opiate-receptor blockade. Although it is still commonly used in emergency rooms to treat opiate overdose, naltrexone is beginning to surpass naloxone for use in the clinical treatment of opiate addiction. Naltrexone is structurally similar to naloxone, but it can be administered orally and is longer lasting. Rapid detoxification is possible under general anesthesia or sedation. The procedure is followed by daily oral doses of naltrexone for up to 12 months or by placement of a naltrexone implant in the lower abdomen or the posterior. Naltrexone is marketed under the trade name Revia, and the extended-release version is marketed as Vivitrol.

Recently, the efficacy of rapid detoxification for long-term opiate dependence management has been questioned. Some argue that rapid detoxification has been misrepresented as a one-time cure for opiate dependence, when it is only the first step in the rehabilitation process. It is also 10 times more expensive than traditional detoxification regimens. In addition, opiate receptors continue to have heightened sensitivity for a period following therapy, during which patients are at high risk for opiate overdose.

WHAT IS THE HISTORY OF OPIATE ADDICTION AND TREATMENT IN THE UNITED STATES?

In the 19th century, most opium in the United States was imported from Southeast Asia and China. It was inexpensive and sold legally throughout the country. By the 1830s, morphine, an opium derivative, was produced legally in Germany, Great Britain, and the United States. Often prescribed to alleviate chronic pain and stress, and sometimes recommended as treatment for chronic alcoholism, opiates were widely available as patent medicines from physicians, pharmacies, grocery stores, and general stores, as well as through the mail. During and after the Civil War, morphine was increasingly used to alleviate pain from battlefield injuries. By 1898, heroin was introduced into pharmacies and quickly became the drug of choice for many addicts, many of whom were veterans and women. Although nonmedical use of opiates was common, it was not considered respectable.

In response to the growing number of addicts, opiate treatment clinics opened in the early 1900s. Similar to MMT programs today, some clinics worked toward total abstinence, whereas others worked toward harm reduction and prescribed or dispensed morphine to addicts. By 1923, these clinics were put out of business by the Narcotics Division of the U.S. Treasury Department, which upheld the prevailing public policy that addiction was not a disease and that addicts were therefore not legitimate medical patients.

Claiming that these clinics were promoting drug use and that the treatment was not medically indicated, the Narcotics Division advised physicians to refrain from dispensing or prescribing morphine. This stance was strengthened by an American Medical Association (AMA) resolution opposing ambulatory clinics, and from 1922 to 1963, it was illegal to dispense or prescribe morphine for the treatment of addiction. Physicians who did so were subject to prosecution.

Methadone, a synthetic analgesic, was developed during World War II by I.G. Farbenendustrie in Germany as an alternative to morphine for treating pain. In 1947, a summary of studies reporting the results of animal and human subjects' reactions to the analgesic qualities of an injectable form of methadone appeared in the *Journal of the American Medical Association*, but the summary did not include methadone as a treatment for opiate withdrawal. It was not until 1949 that studies showed methadone to be an effective medication for withdrawing addicts from heroin. By 1950, oral methadone treatment for opiate withdrawal was used in U.S. Public Health Service hospitals. Methadone's specific pharmacokinetic properties in treating opiate dependence were discovered in 1964.

WHAT IS THE SCOPE OF OPIATE ABUSE IN THE UNITED STATES TODAY?

The problem of opiate abuse in the United States today involves both illegal and legal opiates (i.e., prescription drugs). Heroin is the most widely abused illegal opiate in the country. According to the most recent National Survey on Drug Use and Health (NSDUH), an estimated 166,000 Americans (0.1% of the population) were using heroin, and 4.4 million (1.8%) were using opiate pain relievers without a prescription (Office of Applied Studies [OAS], 2005). Therefore, about 1.9% of the American population were abusing illegal or legal opiates in 2004, representing a drug use problem second only to that posed by marijuana abuse.

In 2002 and 2003, an estimated 354,000 (0.2%) Americans aged 12 or older had used a needle to inject heroin, cocaine, methamphetamines, or other stimulants during the past year (OAS, 2003; OAS, 2004). Among this number were 168,000 who had injected heroin. According to 2002 and 2003 NSDUH data, males were twice as likely as females to inject drugs. Treatment Episode Data Set (TEDS) results from 2004 indicate that 63% of primary heroin admissions reported injection as the mode of use, a percentage not significantly changed from previous years but greatly reduced from the 77% rate reported in 1992 (SAMHSA, 2006). This reduction in the injection rate reported among primary heroin abusers seeking treatment may be attributed to the increase in heroin inhalation. In 2004, 32% of heroin abusers seeking treatment reported inhaling the drug, up from 20% in 1992. About 2% of heroin abusers reported smoking the drug in 2004. Although the trend away from heroin injection seems stable, if not steady, Neaigus et al. (2006) cautioned that several factors may induce a noninjecting user of the drug to turn—or return—to injecting. These factors include a history of injecting; homelessness; adaptation to differences in heroin quality, purity, and availability; increases in the price of heroin; dependence on the drug; drug treatment status; periods of personal trauma or traumatic events; attitudes about the social status of injectors; degree of fear of HIV/AIDS; and degree of comfort with or fear of injecting. Social network influence (particularly from friends, acquaintances, or family members who already inject) may also facilitate a shift to injecting among noninjecting heroin users, placing these users and their sexual partners at greater risk for infection with the hepatitis B and C viruses (HBV and HVC), HIV, and other diseases.

In 2004, an estimated 118,000 Americans had used heroin for the first time within the past 12 months. The average age of first use among recent heroin initiators was 24.4. The 2004 Partnership Attitude Tracking Study (PATS) indicated that few 7th- to 12th-grade teens (4%) had tried heroin (Partnership for a Drug-Free America, 2005). However, about 1 in 7 (16%) teens reported that a close friend had tried the drug. This number is significantly higher than the number from 1998 reports. Taken together with teens' declining recognition of the risks of using heroin (as reported in the PATS over multiple years), this finding could indicate an imminent expansion of heroin use from the young adult population, where its prevalence rate is currently the highest, into the adolescent population.

TEDS data show that treatment admissions for primary heroin abuse increased from 13% of all admissions in 1994 to a peak of 16% in 2001, then fell to 14% in 2004, when the proportion of admissions for primary heroin abuse exceeded that for primary cocaine abuse for the sixth consecutive year. The average age at admission to treatment was 36. About two-thirds (68%) of these admissions were male, half were White (50%), a quarter were African American (24%), and a quarter were Hispanic (23%).

The nonmedical or recreational use of legal pharmaceutical opiates is far more common than the use of illegal opiates in the United States. Opiates other than heroin—such as opium, morphine, codeine, hydrocodone, and oxycodone—are commonly prescribed as pain-relieving medications, but they may be abused, resulting in addiction or dependence. The 2004 NSDUH estimate of 4.4 million current nonprescription opiate users tells only part of the story. In 2002, almost 30 million Americans aged 12 or older (13%) had used prescription pain relievers nonmedically at least once in their lifetime, according to NSDUH estimates. Drug Abuse Warning Network (DAWN) data for 2002 indicate that prescription opiate abuse was involved in 16% of all drug abuse–related emergency department visits, a significant increase over the rates from previous years. NSDUH data show significant increases in lifetime prevalence of use from 2003 to 2004 in several categories of pain relievers among Americans aged 18 to 25. Increases in pain reliever use were statistically significant for Vicodin, Lortab, or Lorcet (from 15.0% to 16.5%); Percocet, Percodan, or Tylox (from 7.8% to 8.7%); hydrocodone products (from 16.3% to 17.4%); OxyContin (from 3.6% to 4.3%); and oxycodone products (from 8.9% to 10.1%). Data for 2004 and early 2005 from predominantly urban sites, as reported by the National Institute on Drug Abuse's (NIDA) Community Epidemiology Work Group (CEWG), suggest the involvement of opiates other than heroin in many deaths (CEWG, 2006). As described in Appendix A and shown by TEDS data, prescription opiates are generally administered orally but may be inhaled or injected.

According to NSDUH 2004 data, the drug category with the largest number of recent initiators was pain relievers used nonmedically. Approximately 2.4 million Americans were estimated to have abused prescription opiates for the first time within the past 12 months—about 20 times the number of heroin initiators in the same period. As noted by CEWG, the impetus to initiate prescription opiate abuse may be the limited availability of high-quality (i.e., pure) heroin in some areas; in other areas, it may be that these drugs are seen as a safe alternative to heroin. The average age for initiating nonmedical use of pain relievers is 23.3, suggesting that younger individuals are abusing these drugs. Accordingly, 2004 PATS data indicate the abuse of a variety of prescription and over-the-counter drugs by 7th- to 12th-grade students. Approximately 1 in 5 teenagers had abused a pain reliever to get high. In 2004, about 1 in 5 teens (18%) reported nonmedical use of Vicodin, and 1 in 10 (10%) reported abuse of OxyContin. Only 48% of teens perceived "great risk" in using prescription drugs nonmedically. Among 12- to 13-year-olds in the 2004 NSDUH sample, nonmedical use of prescription drugs (including opiates) was more common than use of marijuana or inhalants. Combined, the rates of lifetime use of Vicodin and OxyContin for teens in the PATS data set were higher than those of any other drug class except marijuana, prompting the Partnership for a Drug-Free America to label this group of teens "Generation Rx" (Partnership for a Drug-Free America, 2005). These data support anecdotal evidence that some teens take assortments of prescription drugs at parties (the Palm Beach County Substance Abuse Coalition, 2005).

TEDS data show that treatment admissions for primary abuse of opiates other than heroin increased from 1% of all admissions in 1994 to 3% in 2004. These users were generally younger and more likely than heroin users to be entering treatment for the first time. The average age at admission for these nonheroin opiate users was 34 years. Just over half (53%) of primary nonheroin opiate admissions are male; most (89%) are White. From 1992 to 2002, increases in treatment admission rates for abuse of narcotic pain relievers occurred at all levels of urbanization and were greatest in more rural areas. NSDUH data from 2002 to 2003 indicate that users of nonheroin opiates by themselves or in combination with heroin were more likely to report yearly household incomes above $20,000 than were their counterparts who used heroin alone.

Clearly, the scope of opiate abuse in the United States is broad and cuts across boundaries of age, gender, race, and social class. This abuse appears to be a growing trend, particularly among youth.

HOW IS INJECTING DRUG USE ASSOCIATED WITH HEPATITIS AND HIV?

Injecting drug use has long been associated with opiate abuse and is an established risk factor for transmission of blood-borne pathogens, especially HBV, HCV, and HIV. Despite the availability of vaccination against HBV, hepatitis B outbreaks remain frequent among injecting drug users (IDUs). The hepatitis C vaccine is still in trials, and HCV infection is common in

IDU communities. In some MMT programs, as many as 90% of admissions have tested positive for HCV (Tennant, 2001). IDUs may also suffer from alcohol abuse, causing weakened liver condition and thereby exacerbating their rates of HCV. Despite the recognition of elevated rates of hepatitis among IDUs and the higher transmissibility of these viruses, drug users— even those in MMT programs—continue to be underscreened for HBV and HCV, relative to HIV (Hagan, Thiede, & Des Jarlais, 2005; Heimer et al., 2002; Pugatch, Anderson, O'Connell, Elson, & Stein, 2006).

In most of Europe, North Africa, and the Middle East, and in parts of Asia, injecting drug use appears to be the predominant mode of HIV transmission. About 20% of American males and 27% to 34% of American females living with HIV/AIDS in 2004 acquired it through drug injection. The majority of perinatally acquired HIV in the United States can be traced to a parent who was an IDU. Although estimated numbers of HIV/AIDS cases and AIDS-related deaths have decreased among IDUs in the United States since 2000, survival rates after AIDS diagnosis continue to be lowest among males and females who inject drugs. IDUs are at significant risk for infection with any of these viruses. Infection with two or more viruses can seriously complicate the treatment of any single infection.

The risks from injecting drug use are both parenteral (i.e., related to the direct sharing of injection equipment and indirect sharing of ancillary equipment) and sexual. Direct sharing involves using the same needles and syringes that others use to inject drugs. This often occurs because of a lack of access to clean syringes and needles, laws against carrying syringes, and prevailing social and behavioral norms among IDUs. Despite a general consensus among HIV researchers about the harm-reducing effects of needle exchange and syringe exchange programs (NEPs and SEPs), such programs remain relatively uncommon in the United States. In 2002, only 184 U.S. programs were officially active (though more may have worked underground to provide IDUs with sterile supplies), funded by state and city governments, private foundations, and individual donors. The general ambivalence of the American public toward this kind of harm-reduction strategy, however, has meant that NEPs and SEPs remain underfunded and unavailable even in some of the largest cities in the United States.

At the same time, several laws and regulations restrict IDUs' ability or willingness to obtain and carry clean injection equipment. In 2002, 47 states, the District of Columbia, and the Virgin Islands had drug paraphernalia laws that established criminal penalties for, among other things, the sale, distribution, or possession of any item used to administer illegal drugs, including syringes. In the same year, eight states had laws that prohibited dispensing or possessing syringes without a valid medical prescription. Where NEPs or SEPs are available, injectors may be concerned about police activities. They may also worry about being identified as IDUs by members of the community. Even in circumstances with ready access to sterile injecting equipment and where law enforcement is not a concern, IDUs may decide to share syringes or needles or reuse equipment improperly. For example, Mark et al. (2006) reported that one-third of IDUs who participated in Philadelphia needle exchange, detoxification, and MMT programs during the late 1990s continued to share needles during or after participation. The persistence of sharing may be related to a host of factors, including social and behavioral norms about the practice of mutual injection, the presence of relationships outside of drug partnering (especially romantic or sexual involvement), perceptions of relative HIV risk (especially within closed networks of injectors; Unger et al., in press), and convenience. Heimer and Abdala (2000) showed that HIV-1 might survive in used syringes for more than 6 weeks, presenting a significant threat of transmission to any injector who uses them after a seropositive IDU. This viability and the continued tendency toward sharing among a segment of the IDU population has led to the presence of HBV, HCV, and HIV in many MMT patients.

Because of extensive AIDS prevention programs in the United States, needle sharing among IDUs has become more taboo, and practices of cleaning or using new syringes and needles have become more common. The sharing of ancillary injection equipment (i.e., the cooker, cotton, and rinse water), however, remains prevalent. Hagan et al. (2005) suggested that more than half of IDUs reported recent sharing of cookers or cotton. In the Philadelphia study described by Mark et al. (2006; noted above), two-thirds of the study cohort shared injection works during or after participation in treatment. As with the direct sharing of needles and syringes, the indirect sharing of other injection equipment may be linked to a host of factors, including social and behavioral norms and perceptions of the relatively low disease risk posed by this kind of sharing. Despite this perceived low risk, indirect sharing of ancillary equipment has been implicated in the transmission of HBV, HCV, and HIV.

Other risks associated particularly with HIV transmission—but also with HBV and, to a lesser extent, HCV transmission—from IDUs may occur through impairment and unprotected sexual encounters with seropositive IDU partners. Strathdee and Patterson (2006) showed that available data may not accurately demonstrate the impact of injecting drug use on the global spread of HIV/AIDS, as these estimates do not account for sexual transmission associated with having sex with a partner who injects drugs. As early as the mid-1990s, U.S. estimates indicated that 80% of HIV-infected adult heterosexuals who did not inject drugs had been infected by sexual contact with HIV-infected IDUs (Holmberg, 1996). Similar risks are present for noninjecting men who have sex with men (MSM) whose sexual partners are IDUs, compounding the risks presented by MSM activity alone. The noninjecting sex partners of IDUs remain a relatively hidden population in the HIV literature.

Further, knowledge of positive HIV status does not ensure safer sex practices among IDUs. In a Baltimore study, 57% of HIV-positive IDUs reported having had unprotected sex within the past 90 days, 16.4% with HIV-negative partners (Latkin, Forman-Hoffman, D'Souza, & Knowlton, 2004). Unprotected sex may occur more frequently in injector communities, particularly when accompanied by drug use. Impairment may reduce willingness or ability to implement safer sex strategies (e.g., condom use), while increasing the drive to have sex. It may lead IDUs to participate in sexual activities in which they would not otherwise participate. In addition to more frequent incidents of unprotected sex, the trading of sex for drugs or money (often used to buy drugs, but also for basic needs) and sex with multiple partners at one time are commonly reported by IDUs. Both practices have been linked to elevated HIV risk.

A final—and far less publicized—link between injecting drug use and HIV risk involves the lack of adherence to ARV treatment to suppress viral replication in HIV-positive IDUs. Vlahov and Celentano (2006) pointed to the lower use of ARV drugs by active IDUs, which might be linked to the lower socioeconomic status of many IDUs, lack of access to regular health care, and the resulting tendency of HIV-infected IDUs to seek medical attention significantly later in the course of the disease, when ARV treatment might no longer be helpful. Average lower use may also be linked to doctors' concerns about IDU patients' capacity to adhere to ARV; doctors may be reluctant to initiate ARV therapy with these patients. ARV adherence may be difficult for IDUs, as factors commonly found in injecting communities (e.g., mental illness, depression, homelessness) have been negatively correlated with adherence. Further, injecting drug use can impair awareness of the necessary schedules for most ARV regimens. Poor adherence to ARV regimens may lead to incomplete viral suppression in HIV-positive IDUs and increase the potential for development of medication-resistant strains, maintaining or increasing the infection risk posed to the injecting and sexual partners of those IDUs. Nonuse of ARV drugs, however, is certain to increase this risk. Overall, the evidence linking IDU and HIV, both directly and indirectly, is staggering. Although alternative modes of opiate administration have increased in recent years (e.g., oral or inhaling), opiate use remains strongly linked to IDU and thus strongly linked to hepatitis and HIV.

DO COMMUNITIES SUPPORT MMT?

Concerns about the placement of MMT programs divide communities. People who support MMT in theory might protest the opening of an MMT clinic in their neighborhood. Some municipalities have zoning ordinances that prohibit the opening of drug treatment clinics within a certain distance of schools, parks, cultural areas, churches, or residential neighborhoods. Recent court cases over MMT clinic locations have underscored the desire of unwilling neighbors to implement such zoning ordinances. The most common argument against establishing MMT programs is that once patients leave the clinics, they can again become drug users and are then likely to be involved in criminal activities in the communities where the programs are located. However, MMT-related crime statistics contradict this assertion (Nurco, 1990). Another common (and related) argument is that the presence of MMT clinics brings more drug users into an area. Although this argument may be supportable in some areas, it shows a general unwillingness to recognize the presence of drug users in one's own community. Years of drug research have revealed that drug abuse is as much a problem in communities where it is assumed to be absent as it is in those where it is unequivocally recognized. The prevalent and persistent opposition that communities demonstrate is a significant barrier to expanding access to MMT.

HOW DOES MMT ACT AS A HARM-REDUCTION STRATEGY?

Harm reduction focuses on minimizing the negative outcomes of continued substance abuse. It incorporates a spectrum of strategies, ranging from safer use education to managed use to abstinence. Harm reduction aims to address the conditions and contexts of substance use while addressing the drug use itself. MMT functions as a harm-reduction strategy by decreasing the cravings for opiates and, in turn, decreasing the frequency of injecting drug use and the possibility of sharing injecting equipment, thereby reducing the potential negative consequences of injecting drug use. Methadone works by providing chemical signals similar to those derived from other opiates, while avoiding the disorienting euphoria associated with these drugs. The length of time that a patient subscribes to MMT varies among treatment centers and patients. In 2003, just over one-fifth of the MMT centers in the United States had policies encouraging withdrawal from methadone within 12 months; more than half, however, permitted patients to remain in MMT indefinitely (Levine, Reif, Lee, Ritter, & Horgan, 2004).

MMT is not a cure for opiate dependence, per se, but rather a therapy that allows a patient to function normally while giving counseling and other treatments a chance to work. In 2003, 95% of MMT programs taught risk-reduction skills and offered HIV antibody testing and counseling, 89% offered tuberculosis (TB) screening, and 50% offered employment counseling and training. Some programs—particularly those run by private, nonprofit organizations—offered child care and transportation to the treatment center (Levine et al., 2004). Hepatitis screening and counseling are becoming more common in MMT programs. The ability to provide all of these services in one location, coupled with the mental clarity provided by methadone itself, has made MMT the most effective treatment for opiate dependence to date.

MMT has been associated with significant reductions in HIV, HBV, and HCV transmission. A review of methadone studies from the early 1980s to 2003 (Gowing, Farrell, Bornemann, Sullivan, & Ali, 2006) reported significant reductions in HIV risk among drug users with a history of sustained MMT. The studies demonstrated a consistent decrease in the proportion of participants who reported injecting, the frequency of injection, the sharing of ancillary equipment, and drug-related HIV risk scores. The data suggest a lower likelihood of multiple sex partners and exchanges of sex for drugs or money. Rates of unprotected sex seem less subject to change under MMT. In a study of MMT combined with behavioral interventions, however, the number of patients reporting unprotected sex declined by 88% under the influence of the combination therapy (Schroeder et al., 2006). All of these reductions in HIV risk behavior should be seen as reductions in the risk of HBV and HCV transmission as well. Further, MMT seems to be linked to a lower rate of progression to AIDS among HIV-positive clients (Gowing et al., 2006). This lower progression rate may reflect the reduction of risk behaviors, as noted above, but also indicates an association between participation in MMT and adherence to ARV regimens (Palepu et al., in press).

In addition, MMT has been linked to reductions in crime-related activities. In communities where MMT programs are established, criminal behavior may be reduced by as much as 50% (NIDA, 1999). These reductions reflect not only arrests for possession and use of drugs, but also drug-related robbery, burglary, and larceny. MMT also has an effect on employment. In qualitative interviews, MMT clients have reported that methadone has allowed them to concentrate on work (Zule & Desmond, 1998), perhaps because methadone can be taken once a day rather than necessitating use throughout the day (as with other opiates) and perhaps because it does not generally produce a disorienting high. For some reason, communities with MMT programs may experience employment increases of up to 40% (NIDA, 1999). MMT's generally positive outcomes go beyond improvements in clients' health status, significantly affecting the social and economic circumstances of clients' everyday lives.

Moreover, the controversy surrounding MMT involves concerns about the philosophy of drug maintenance treatment. Such philosophical concerns are often tied to broader concerns about the acceptability of harm-reduction strategies as opposed to strategies designed to produce total abstinence from drug use. Skeptics often see the "any positive change" message of harm reduction as too permissive in a nation committed to the "just say no" message for drug use. For these opponents, harm reduction allows for a continuation of the drug problem rather than providing a solution. Many politicians, public health practitioners, and even IDUs themselves view MMT as a way to replace one addiction with another. The maintenance dose of methadone becomes the new drug of addiction for MMT patients, who are therefore not truly drug free. Debate about this kind of drug replacement therapy can be found even inside MMT programs; where some physicians prefer to use methadone as an intermediate step to total abstinence and others prefer to allow patients to remain on methadone indefinitely. Unfortunately, while this philosophical controversy continues both inside MMT programs and in the broader public arena, the social, political, and economic barriers to greater MMT success are unlikely to be removed.

CHAPTER 2—The Effectiveness of Methadone and the History of Regulation

MMT is subject to complex regulatory constraints. In this chapter, we review the evidence of MMT's effectiveness, including prior studies of the quality of services. We then discuss the ways in which it has been regulated in the United States, ending with a review of the accreditation model.

IS MMT EFFECTIVE?

MMT is the primary form of opiate dependence treatment in the United States. The first well-publicized evaluation of its effectiveness was a research project at Rockefeller University whose results were published in 1965 by Dole and Nyswander. This study, which used oral methadone to treat dependence, found that once the optimal dose was achieved, patients could be maintained on a steady dose to prevent abstinence symptoms. Following this nationally recognized study, methadone gained acceptance as an effective treatment for opiate dependence, and the number of MMT programs began to increase across the country.

While clinical trials continued to assess the effectiveness of methadone to treat opiate dependence, the next significant advance occurred in 1991 when Ball and Ross published results from a large-scale analysis of 507 continuing patients and 126 new admissions to six MMT programs in New York, Philadelphia, and Baltimore. Conducted during the mid-1980s, the Ball and Ross study was the most detailed examination of MMT programs to date. Although this study found differences in the effectiveness of MMT to be a function of the severity of patients' conditions, the number of services provided during treatment, and particularly the dosages (higher dosages produced better outcomes), the results showed significant reductions in heroin and nonopiate drug use as well as in crime. A significant number of addicts continued using heroin when their daily methadone dose was less than 70 mg, whereas most patients receiving more than 70 mg a day stopped using heroin. The prevalence of injecting drug use for the 388 patients who remained in MMT decreased from 81% at admission to 29% after 4 years of treatment.

In addition to detailing the effectiveness of MMT, the Ball and Ross study revealed wide disparities in treatment practices, such as drug screening, urine testing requirements, staffing credentials, methadone dosage levels, restrictions on take-home doses, types and intensity of rehabilitation services offered, and discharge policies. MMT programs also differed sharply in the provision of medical care for their patients, use of ancillary psychotherapeutic medications (e.g., antidepressants and antipsychotics), uniformity of rule enforcement, counselors' caseloads, psychiatric input, quality of in-service training, and physician facilities.

Characteristics of more effective programs included year-to-year staff stability, higher patient retention rates, adequate methadone doses, high rates of scheduled attendance, and a close and consistent relationship between staff and patients. With regard to treatment services, Ball and Ross found that both staff and patients viewed counseling as a key element in the MMT rehabilitative process. The long-term rehabilitative aspects of MMT programs were found to be more important in successful treatment than short-term pharmacological issues. Programs that provided a high level of treatment services to patients were associated with decreases in heroin, cocaine, and injecting drug use, along with decreases in criminal behavior. The lack of randomization of patients in this study, however, made generalization of these findings difficult.

In the early 1990s, methadone effectiveness was again demonstrated through NIDA-funded research examining the public health benefits of MMT (Metzger et al., 1995; Wechsberg et al., 1993). NIDA studies compared the rates of AIDS risk behaviors (particularly injecting drug use and needle sharing) between samples of opiate addicts in MMT and addicts not in treatment. Metzger et al. found that at baseline, 13% of patients in MMT were HIV-positive, compared with 21% of the opiate addicts who were not in treatment. Over a 3-year period, an additional 5% of patients in MMT became infected with HIV; however, these were only patients who dropped out of treatment. Among out-of-treatment opiate addicts, an additional 26%

became infected with HIV over the same period. Although the findings do not show that methadone was the causal agent generating the differences in infection rates, they do suggest that participation in MMT was at least one factor in the reduction of AIDS risk. Further evidence of the effectiveness of MMT is provided in peer-reviewed journals from 1988 to 1999 (Phillips et al., 1995; Zaric et al., 2000).

The National Treatment Improvement Evaluation Study (NTIES), a congressionally mandated 5-year longitudinal study of the impact of drug and alcohol treatment, surveyed thousands of patients in hundreds of treatment units nationally (Gerstein, 1997). The study received public support from the Substance Abuse and Mental Health Services Administration (SAMHSA) through a Center for Substance Abuse Treatment (CSAT) demonstration grant funding program in 1990 and 1991. The study was designed to address two questions: how much MMT is required to achieve successful outcomes, and to what extent will favorable outcomes persist following termination from treatment? The results indicated that MMT is effective in reducing heroin use and supporting positive treatment outcomes. The NTIES study provided support for an expansion of MMT, aftercare services for MMT patients, and ancillary services, such as transportation and child care to support retention in treatment.

As the findings from these studies and many others show, with appropriate dosage, MMT can be effective in treating opiate dependence and enabling patients to reduce heroin use, drug-seeking criminal behaviors, and HIV risk. Moreover, a large proportion of patients in MMT programs are able to function more effectively in the workplace and in other social relationships while supported by the treatment services they receive from MMT programs.

WHAT IS THE HISTORY OF MMT REGULATION IN THE UNITED STATES?

After World War I, opiate dependence continued in urban areas but gradually shifted from European immigrants to African Americans and Hispanics who moved to northern industrial cities as Europeans moved into suburban areas. Attitudes changed from compassion and support for opiate-dependent females and veterans to disdain toward and stigmatization of poor and minority addicts in inner-city ghettos.

The first national response to the changing image of the addict occurred as an act of Congress. The Harrison Narcotic Act of 1914 was passed to fulfill the country's obligations to uphold the international agreement of the 1912 Hague Convention.

The Harrison Act was not originally written as a prohibition law but as a means to regulate the manufacture, distribution, and prescription of opiates, cocaine, and their derivatives and to decrease opium trade with Southeast Asia and China. The Act made it illegal to possess any of these drugs unless licensed by the Internal Revenue Bureau of the Treasury Department. All manufacturers, pharmacists, and physicians had to be licensed and keep records on narcotics. The Act allowed physicians to prescribe narcotics only for what were considered to be legitimate medical purposes in the course of professional practice. It did not allow prescription of narcotics for mainte-nance, because the Treasury Department did not categorize addiction as a disease, and addicts were not seen as legitimate patients.

The position of the Treasury Department was upheld in 1919 by a Supreme Court ruling, which in effect outlawed opiate dependence mainte-nance treatment. This interpretation of the Harrison Act led to an era of strong narcotics regulation.

In later years, the incidence of addiction and crimes related to addiction rose dramatically in urban areas. The federal government responded between 1936 and 1938 by opening two U.S. Public Health Service hospitals for the treatment of addiction. Located in Lexington, Kentucky, and in Fort Worth, Texas, the hospitals were the principal resources for addiction treatment in the United States until the 1960s (Kreek, 2000).

Both the legal and medical professions in the United States were upset by the rise in heroin addiction and its associated social, criminal, and medical consequences. In 1956, the Joint Committee of the American Bar Association and AMA were joined to review the problem. The committee issued a report in 1958 that recommended the establishment of an outpatient clinic to prescribe narcotics on a controlled experimental basis. In 1963, President Kennedy's Advisory Commission on Narcotic and Drug Abuse also recommended that research be conducted to determine the effectiveness of dispensing narcotics in outpatient facilities.

In the early 1970s, White House staff under President Nixon commissioned the National Institute of Mental Health (NIMH), in collaboration with several other federal offices, to provide policy and program recommendations for initiatives to respond to the increase in heroin addiction. At the same time, White House staff invited comments from a nongovernmental advisory group of professionals in the field of substance abuse. The NIMH-led group recommended that methadone be further investigated as a treatment modality. The nonfederal advisory group proposed a strategy to rapidly expand all forms of treatment, including MMT. In response to the policy recommendations, President Nixon named Dr. Jerome Jaffe as the Director of the Special Action Office for Drug Abuse Prevention (SAODAP). One of the early goals of this office was to promulgate Food and Drug Administration (FDA) regulations that would govern the use of methadone to treat opiate dependence (FDA, 1972).

To further support the work being conducted by FDA, legislation established the Alcohol, Drug Abuse, and Mental Health Administration (ADAMHA) within the National Institutes of Health (NIH) in 1974. As a successor to both SAODAP and ADAMHA, Congress created SAMHSA in 1992. This new legislation defined SAMHSA as an agency separate and distinct from NIH. With the creation of SAMHSA, Congress transferred drug abuse demand reduction services from NIDA to SAMHSA, leaving research activities with NIDA (Harrison, Bachenheimer, & Inciardi, 1995).

In the late 1970s, FDA and NIDA jointly promulgated standards for MMT programs. These standards were developed as a means to regulate the safety and improve the effectiveness of MMT programs through a formal approval and monitoring process. The regulations created state authorities to participate in the process of approving and evaluating programs. However, early regulations were criticized by practitioners as interfering in the practice of medicine, and both federal and state regulations were revised several times.

Almost since the inception of these regulations, there has been strong criticism of the regulatory process governing the provision of MMT. The

Narcotic Addiction Treatment Act of 1974 (NATA) further defined MMT by requiring that all treatment programs register with the Drug Enforcement Agency (DEA), which became responsible for monitoring and preventing methadone diversion (NATA, 1974). Concurrently, DHHS was given primary authority for determining standards for MMT and providing oversight to ensure that these standards were met. The final FDA regulations remained substantively unchanged for more than 25 years, despite several major efforts to address concerns regarding the regulatory structure under FDA.

WHAT IS THE QUALITY OF MMT SERVICES?

As clinical and evaluative research examined and supported the effectiveness of MMT, federal agencies began to shift focus and concentrate on the quality of MMT services. In 1988, Thomas D'Aunno at the Institute for Social Research conducted a study of patients in MMT units (D'Aunno et al., 1999). One aim of the study was to provide policy makers and treatment managers with information about the type and amount of services patients were receiving in outpatient drug abuse treatment units in the United States. Another aim was to examine the extent to which differences in both client characteristics and key organizational factors were related to differences in medical and social services that patients received in treatment units. The findings indicated that variations across MMT programs included client characteristics, service intensity, and dosage. Staffing patterns were shown to have little relationship to MMT practices.

As a result of findings from these studies by D'Aunno, Ball and Ross, and other researchers, Congress commissioned the General Accounting Office (GAO; now called the Government Accountability Office) to gather information on MMT using a case study approach. The goal of the GAO study was to provide a report to the Select Committee on Narcotics Abuse and Control regarding the quality of MMT. GAO found that policies, goals, and practices varied greatly among MMT programs and reported that no programs currently evaluated the effectiveness of the treatment they provided. Further, GAO reported that most MMT programs prescribed average methadone doses below the minimum amount recommended for effective treatment and that programs varied widely in urine testing procedures; nine programs conducted no drug testing. Programs also varied with regard to discharge criteria. Overall, nearly half of the programs examined could not demonstrate the delivery of effective MMT. Patient outcomes varied, and many patients reported continued use of heroin.

The Methadone Treatment Quality Assurance System (MTQAS), funded by NIDA, was created in response to the GAO report (Czechowicz et al., 1997; Ducharme & Luckey, 2000). The project was charged with developing and testing a performance-based measurement system for MMT programs, and MTQAS accordingly identified factors critical to successful systems. The MTQAS methodology differentiated performance on a number of independent dimensions, providing critical clarification on where improvements were most needed in a given program. The project provided evidence that a performance-based feedback system could be implemented at the state level. At the conclusion of the project, however, only three of the seven states involved indicated plans to continue participating in MTQAS.

In separate studies, researchers evaluated how counseling and psychosocial services provided during MMT contributed to patient outcomes (Friedmann et al., 2000; McLellan et al., 1993). McLellan et al. found results indicating that although an adequate methadone dosage level significantly reduced levels of heroin use, greater reductions in heroin use were obtained through adjunctive counseling and other services. This study also showed that medication in conjunction with counseling and other psychosocial services enabled greater social rehabilitation.

The Alcohol and Drug Services Study (ADSS) built on SAMHSA research completed in the early 1990s. Sponsored by OAS, ADSS was designed to collect information on the characteristics of substance abuse treatment facilities and their patients (Levine et al., 2002). ADSS was also designed to study relationships among facility characteristics, treatment services, and patients in treatment. SAMHSA was interested in developing better estimates of patient length of stay and the costs of treatment, and in describing the post treatment status of patients.

ADSS found that 6% of the estimated 688 facilities across the country offered outpatient MMT during 1996. These outpatient MMT facilities were typically larger than facilities that did not offer outpatient MMT, had more private for-profit ownership, relied more on self-payment, were located in larger metropolitan areas, and were more likely to be licensed and accredited by state public health agencies. These facilities reported fewer treatment and support services than other types of care facilities and had higher patient-to-staff outpatient ratios. ADSS estimated that MMT programs were serving more than 150,000 patients, or 14% of all patients in the treatment system. The study reported that many MMT patients had multiple problems and were more likely than other patients in treatment to be older and receiving disability benefits.

Overall, ADSS found that MMT programs provided a mean of 11 treatment services. ADSS also reported that withdrawal policies had changed; 52% of facilities permitted patients to remain in MMT for an unlimited time, and 78% of facilities discouraged methadone withdrawal within a year of treatment. Facilities dispensing higher dosages were more likely to have liberal withdrawal policies. Facilities that encouraged withdrawal within a year had a mean daily methadone dosage of less than 60 mg. The majority of facilities offered HIV/AIDS education, counseling, and support; TB screening; and employment counseling or training. Private, for-profit facilities were least likely to offer HIV/AIDS support services, transportation, and child care support services. Publicly owned facilities offered the most services and discouraged withdrawal but tended to provide lower methadone dosages. The study concluded that the provision of treatment services varied greatly across MMT programs, but programs were providing high-quality services through higher dosages and through less required early withdrawal.

By the mid-1990s, the topics of MMT quality and patient outcomes had risen to the federal level, with mixed evidence from research. MMT continued to demonstrate benefits for the patient population; however, the variability of services provided within the field was cause for concern.

HOW HAS MMT REGULATION CHANGED IN THE UNITED STATES?

Outdated federal regulations, combined with a heightened focus on accountability and quality in the late 1980s and early 1990s, prompted questions regarding the level of care provided by MMT programs. The 1990 GAO report revealed not only wide disparity across MMT programs but also minimal federal oversight of MMT (GAO, 1990). Specifically, GAO observed that although FDA and NIDA had responsibility for regulating MMT, these agencies provided little oversight for the programs. Federal regulations did not establish performance standards, such as the percentage of patients no longer using heroin. GAO also observed that although official FDA policy was to inspect each program once every 2 years, at the time of the GAO visits, none of the programs had been inspected within the previous 5 years. The GAO report recommended that results-oriented standards be developed to set expectations for MMT programs and to provide a basis for assessing treatment effectiveness according to the National Drug Control Strategy.

To investigate the effectiveness of the MMT regulatory system, NIDA, SAMHSA, and the Office of the Assistant Secretary for Health funded a 2-year Institute of Medicine (IOM) study of the current regulations, including enforcement issues, quality of treatment, and diversion (Rettig & Yarmolinsky, 1995). IOM concluded that the current regulations had little effect on the quality of treatment provided in MMT programs. In particular, the report emphasized the need to balance process-oriented regulations with clinical practice guidelines and quality assurance systems. IOM found that enforceable federal standards were needed, not for medical reasons but to prevent substandard or unethical practices and to maintain community support. Therefore, IOM recommended that the regulations governing MMT be reduced in scope to be less regimented and thus allow more clinical judgment and professional discretion in MMT treatment. Clinical practice guidelines, according to IOM, would ensure that clinical discretion was exercised in a sound manner and would serve to improve the quality of treatment services.

As MMT became recognized as an effective treatment modality, the substance abuse treatment field was evolving. The emphasis on the process of substance abuse treatment was superseded by a focus on the outcome of substance abuse treatment. Performance measurement, quality assurance, and accountability became critical factors in monitoring substance abuse services. These changes brought a new focus to the regulation and service delivery of opiate dependence treatment; public protection and validation of

MMT were no longer driving the delivery and regulation of treatment for opiate dependence. Instead, the new focus was on performance measurement and outcomes, resulting in the precedence of service delivery over process. This dramatically changing environment prompted both the government and clinical entrepreneurs to work toward repealing the FDA regulatory system and substituting a system that would emphasize performance measurement and quality assurance among MMT programs.

The IOM report suggested modifying regulations to encourage comprehensive care for patients, continual reassessment of patient progress and needs, treatment based on clinical practice guidelines, and humane treatment of patients. At the request of the Secretary of DHHS, these recommendations were reviewed by the Interagency Narcotic Treatment and Policy Review Board (INTPRB), a working group originally convened under the Special Action Officer of Drug Abuse Policy (SAODAP).

Based on a review of the IOM recommendations, INTPRB recommended developing an accreditation-based system centered on a core set of federal treatment standards, in conjunction with monitoring treatment programs through private accreditation. INTPRB concluded that this would be both feasible and preferable to the existing system under FDA. A 1997 National Institutes of Health (NIH) consensus panel supported the INTPRB findings and concluded that existing federal and state regulations limited the ability of physicians and other health care professionals to provide high-quality, individualized MMT services to patients and recommended that federal regulations be eliminated.

Following the GAO and IOM reports, as well as the INTPRB recommendations, concerns about the variability in type and quality of services provided in MMT programs could no longer go unaddressed. Recognizing the need to improve quality of care in MMT and better monitor MMT operations, DHHS convened an interagency workgroup to draft revised regulations. CSAT, in collaboration with other federal agencies, convened a consensus panel to develop treatment service guidelines for MMT. The guidelines were developed through a series of meetings with federal and state officials, treatment experts, and patient/consumer advocates. Along with the treatment standards in the revised regulations, these guidelines formed the basis for the new accreditation standards. An overview of the history leading to the new guidelines and current regulatory requirements is presented in Figure 2.1.

WHAT IMPACT DOES THE NEW REGULATORY SYSTEM HAVE ON HOW MMT IS PROVIDED?

With the need for new regulation for MMT clearly documented, the next step was to define guidelines for creating and implementing a new regulatory system for the oversight and delivery of MMT. In December 1996, CSAT convened a special field-based guideline development panel of pharmacotherapy experts to provide content for the process of developing guidelines on providing and evaluating MMT.

As a first step, CSAT created a preliminary outline, which was shared with a resource panel of federal and nonfederal experts. Once the resource panel approved the outline, workgroups were established to take responsibility for developing specific draft treatment standards. An expert review panel was held on January 14, 1998, to provide a secondary review and to further refine the document. In addition, this document was circulated for review and comment to additional treatment experts and federal officials.

The new system calls on SAMHSA-approved accreditation organizations to evaluate MMT programs and to provide specific recommendations for program improvement. Accreditation organizations follow the CSAT guidelines to develop specific MMT accreditation standards for compliance. Below is a list of the guidelines' areas that represent the domains found in the Final Rule, serving to drive the development and revision of accreditation standards and MMT practice and processes (CSAT, 2001):

- administrative organization and responsibilities
- management of facility and clinical environment
- risk management and continuous quality improvement
- professional staff credentials and development
- patient admission criteria
- patient medical and psychosocial assessment

Figure 2.1 Evolution of Regulatory Change in the United States

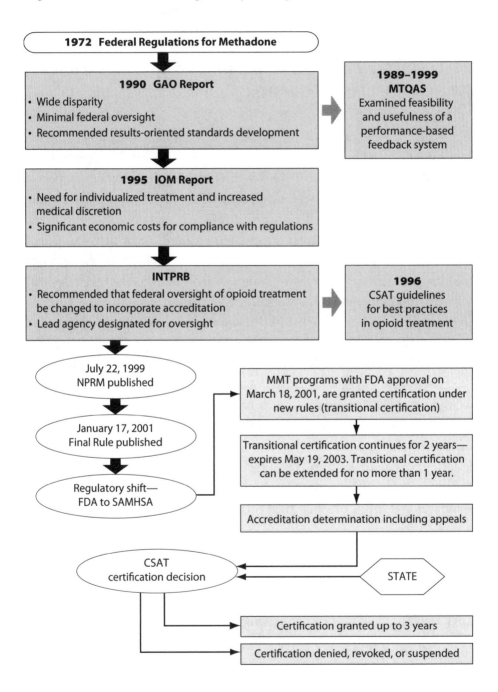

- guidelines for therapeutic dosage
- treatment planning, evaluation of patient progress in treatment, and continuous clinical assessment
- testing for drug use
- unsupervised approved use (take-home medication)
- withdrawal and discharge
- management of concurrent alcohol and polysubstance abuse
- concurrent services
- special considerations
- care of females in treatment
- patients' rights
- record keeping and documentation
- community relations and education
- diversion control

WHY WAS AN EVALUATION OF ACCREDITATION NEEDED?

Changes recommended to the existing FDA regulated system for MMT represented the culmination of research and policy analysis spanning more than a decade. The existing system had remained unchanged for nearly 25 years. For policy change of this magnitude, the federal government depends on evaluation research to assess the impact on the field. In recognition of this need, SAMHSA set aside federal dollars to fund an evaluation study.

SUMMARY

- In addition to reviewing the effectiveness and importance of MMT, this chapter delineates the regulation history and explains how it has shifted in recent years.
- MMT is the primary form of opiate dependence treatment in the United States.

- Dole and Nyswander published on the effectiveness of oral methadone in treating addiction in 1965. This was the first well-publicized example of the effectiveness of methadone in treating addiction.

- Ball and Ross published a detailed examination of MMT programs in 1991. This publication showed significant associated reductions in heroin and nonopiate drug use and crime among MMT patients.

- Research funded by NIDA in the early 1990s demonstrated the public health benefits of MMT by comparing rates of AIDS risk behavior between opiate addicts in MMT and addicts not in treatment. MMT was found to be a factor in reduction of AIDS risk.

- Since the late 1970s, FDA has had regulatory oversight for MMT, and DEA has overseen methadone dispersion and diversion. This regulatory structure has remained substantively unchanged for more than 25 years.

- During the late 1980s and early 1990s, policy makers began to question the quality of MMT. After review, GAO found that policies, goals, and practices varied greatly among MMT programs. GAO also found that most programs prescribed average methadone doses below the minimum amount recommended for effective treatment.

- In 1997, an NIH consensus panel concluded that the existing federal and state regulations limited the ability of physicians and other health professionals to provide MMT services to patients. This panel recommended that federal regulations be changed.

- As a result of the NIH consensus panel recommendations, regulatory oversight of MMT shifted from FDA to DHHS and SAMHSA. DHHS began the process of implementing an accreditation-based regulatory system, and DEA remained responsible for methadone dispersion and diversion oversight.

- The new accreditation-based system follows guidelines developed by CSAT. MMT programs are now expected to comply with these specific guidelines and accreditation standards.

CHAPTER 3—The Accreditation Evaluation Study

The Accreditation Evaluation Study is the largest recent national study of MMT. This chapter reviews its objectives and design and explains how the data were collected and analyzed.

WHAT IS THE ACCREDITATION EVALUATION STUDY?

The Accreditation Evaluation Study (Evaluation Study) is the past decade's largest nationally representative study of MMT. From 1998 through 2001, it examined the processes, barriers, and costs associated with the change from an FDA-regulated system (Rettig & Yarmolinsky, 1995) to a SAMHSA-oversight system supported by an accreditation organization for MMT programs. The Evaluation Study addressed the process of preparing and applying for accreditation and included a comparison of required activities. It was also charged with identifying changes in clinical policies and practices, service accessibility and delivery, and patient characteristics in accredited MMT programs several months after an accreditation site visit. As part of the Evaluation Study, an economic analysis was completed on the program costs of preparing for an initial accreditation site visit.

WHAT WAS THE EVALUATION STUDY'S DESIGN?

The conceptual model of the Evaluation Study proposed to answer one primary policy question: what impact will accreditation and a new SAMHSA-oversight system have on MMT programs and the field of opiate dependence treatment? To answer this question, the study was conducted using an experimental design with a baseline and follow-up measurement of the same constructs within experimental and control sites. The intervention for experimental sites was to prepare for and undergo an accreditation site visit. Most data were captured at two points: baseline and following accreditation. Then the two data sets were compared over time and between experimental and control sites. To most accurately capture the activities and costs associated with preparing for and participating in an accreditation survey, the study collected information from experimental sites while they were preparing for accreditation and from a control group for comparison. Control programs did not undergo an accreditation site visit until after completion of data collection for the Evaluation Study.

The study design was intended to avoid the bias associated with the participatory self-selection of sites that were most interested in obtaining accreditation. By including a control group, the evaluators were able to distinguish between the temporal trends and market influences that affected the larger MMT field during the study period (1998 to 2001) and changes attributable to undergoing the accreditation process.

Initially, the analytic plan called for collecting steady-state baseline measures from all sites approximately 6 to 9 months before an MMT program's accreditation survey and collecting follow-up measures 6 months after completion of the accreditation visit. The plan established comparable data collection dates for control sites. In practice, delays created an 8- to 15-month window between the baseline evaluation site visit and the accreditation survey. A 6- to 8-month window following the accreditation visit was viewed as necessary to allow sites to return to a steady state so that initial impacts of accreditation could be assessed. Comparisons between these two points then yielded information on changes in site operations.

The final analytic design sought to reflect the priorities that emerged from the various governmental activities preceding the regulatory changes. The Evaluation Study, therefore, systematically examined the activities, characteristics of sites, administrative outcomes, and costs related to compliance with the newly defined CSAT guidelines as implemented through the accreditation standard, as well as the impact of accreditation on methadone diversion, program accessibility, patient population served, staff attitudes and behavior, and patient satisfaction.

WHO PARTICIPATED IN THE EVALUATION STUDY?

Fifteen states (Figure 3.1) were selected to participate in the study after meeting one or more of the following criteria: (1) geographic distribution throughout the four U.S. census regions, (2) encompassing a large number of

MMT programs and representing different models of treatment or state regulation, (3) participation in MTQAS from 1989 to 1999, and (4) mandating accreditation or accepted deemed status for licensure or certification. States outside the contiguous United States and states with fewer than four MMT programs were excluded.

Figure 3.1   States Participating in the Accreditation Evaluation Study

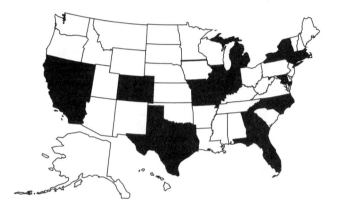

The second stage of the sampling process was program selection. The number of programs selected from each state was designed to be proportional to the overall distribution of MMT programs in each state (i.e., states with the largest number of MMT programs had the largest representation in the sample). For Evaluation Study purposes, sampled programs were the individual MMT unit rather than overall treatment organizations (which may have a single unit or multiple units). This allowed evaluation of the impact of accreditation on individual treatment facilities. All programs within a given state were eligible for selection, except for sites that had a unique structure or current regulatory oversight. MMT programs were excluded from the study if they were a correctional facility, medication dispensing unit, or hospital-based detoxification facility or if they were operated by the Department of Veterans Affairs. These programs were excluded because of their unique structures or regulatory oversight at the time of the study.

The baseline data used in the Evaluation Study were collected from the total number of sites (n=172; Table 3.1). Surveys were administered to a cohort of staff and patients at a program during a site visit.

Table 3.1   Participants from Preaccreditation Site Visit Data Collection

Participant Group	Sample Size
MMT program	172
Staff (nonphysician)	1,414
Physician	244
Patient	6,860

Note: MMT = methadone maintenance treatment.

Research analysts (from RTI International) completed follow-up data collection site visits at 144 of the 172 MMT programs participating in baseline site visits. Follow-up site visits were conducted between April 2000 and July 2001. Twenty sites that participated in the baseline site visits dropped out of the study; five sites were not prepared to complete the accreditation site visit within the study time frame and were recorded as passed over; two sites were identified as residential therapeutic community sites and were determined to be outliers; and one site was excluded because of a group classification error (Table 3.2).

Of the 144 MMT programs that completed follow-up site visits, 104 underwent the accreditation process and are referred to as experimental sites; 40 served as control sites and underwent accreditation after the conclusion of the study. The Commission on Accreditation of Rehabilitation Facilities (CARF; 1998) and the Joint Commission on Accreditation of Healthcare Organizations (JCAHO; 2000) conducted the accreditation site visits.

The purpose of the follow-up site visits was to collect repeated cross-sectional data at a point in time after the accreditation site visits. Follow-up site visits were conducted 6 to 8 months after MMT programs had undergone the accreditation process for experimental programs and during the same time frame for control programs.

Table 3.2   Follow-Up Site Visit Participants

	Number of Sites
Experimental	
Completed baseline survey	128
Dropped out	18
Passed over	5
Outlier dropped from analyses (residential program or therapeutic community)	1
Total experimental sites in follow-up	104
Control	
Completed baseline survey	44
Dropped out	2
Outlier dropped from analyses (residential program or therapeutic community)	1
Group classification error	1
Total control sites in follow-up	40
Total follow-up sites	144

WHAT DATA WERE COLLECTED?

The Evaluation Study researchers began data collection by collecting program-level information such as program name, address, telephone number, initial contact name, and experimental or comparison group assignment. This information was compiled and maintained in a Microsoft Access project database. Each program was assigned to an RTI data collection team whose members were responsible for scheduling and conducting both the pre- and post-accreditation data collection visits. These team members were the primary point of contact between the MMT program and RTI. Once the visit date was scheduled, advance materials were sent to the program director approximately 2 to 4 weeks before the program visit. These materials included the following:

- a cover letter explaining the Evaluation Study and the research commitments required of the program

- a program survey
- two cost questionnaires
- a physician questionnaire

Staff questionnaires, patient questionnaires, and abstraction forms (dosing log, waiting list form, urinalysis log, discharge log) were administered while staff were on-site during a 2-day visit. Data from programs, physicians, patients, and staff were collected using 12 data collection instruments and abstraction forms. The areas of opiate dependence treatment examined were as follows:

- organizational characteristics
- staff characteristics
- patient characteristics
- comprehensiveness of services
- professional discretion
- performance measurement and quality assurance

HOW WERE THE DATA ANALYZED?

Descriptive data analyses were conducted using data collected during the preaccreditation visit with the programs. All estimates used weighted data, allowing results to be generalized to the appropriate population of MMT programs. These baseline statistics provide a comprehensive overview of the field across all study constructs at a time before accreditation.

Individual program data were aggregated to obtain mean values of individual variables and factor scores. Individual variables were either single items from the questionnaires or derived variables obtained by recoding or combining multiple items from the questionnaires. These variables were not standardized but were analyzed using the same significance tests as the factor scores. Factor scores were standardized so that all means were equal to 0 and all standard deviations were equal to 1. In some analyses, factor scores developed during the baseline analyses were used to compare results within and between experimental and control MMT programs.

The final report (CSAT, 2001) developed by RTI for SAMHSA as part of the Evaluation Study contains all data analyses conducted, including (1) descriptive data analyses at baseline, (2) change data analyses comparing pre- and post-data for both experimental and control sites, and (3) all factor analyses. Information presented in this book focuses primarily on descriptive analyses of MMT programs, and we provide an in-depth examination of the characteristics of these programs in the United States during the late 1990s.

HOW DID THE EVALUATION STUDY CHANGE FROM ITS INCEPTION?

The Evaluation Study evolved as the changing field of opiate dependence treatment reacted to recommendations for improving the quality of treatment services. Within the study time frame, there was continued movement toward a regulatory shift from FDA to SAMHSA, and a Proposed Rule addressing this shift was published during data collection. Thus, the Evaluation Study changed in focus from a feasibility study to an impact analysis.

To avoid any misinterpretation of the study findings, it should be understood that the Evaluation Study focused on the impact of accreditation, not on the value of accreditation. It was designed to examine ways to improve the process of accreditation and certification and to determine what characteristics of treatment were affected through the process.

The Evaluation Study was

- a stratified random sample with experimental and control group comparisons;

- designed to collect pretests and post-tests;

- able to identify changes that accreditation may have prompted in clinical policies and practices, service accessibility and delivery, and patient characteristics for MMT;

- able to capture the MMT costs of preparing for, undergoing, and achieving accreditation status; and

- designed to provide estimates of the average MMT costs and labor hours across programs and by key program characteristics, such as size, ownership, and urbanicity.

The Evaluation Study was *not*

- a feasibility study (i.e., it did not attempt to evaluate the worth of an accreditation-based monitoring system, but examined the impact of accreditation on MMT programs);

- historical (i.e., it did not compare FDA activities with the efforts being pursued by the private accrediting bodies engaged in the accreditation project);

- a comparison of accrediting bodies;

- a method of determining diversion;

- a long-term longitudinal study (i.e., it evaluated MMT at two points within a specific, relatively short time frame);

- able to identify and calculate resource use and expenditures for pursuing specific accreditation requirements;

- able to estimate the costs of maintaining accreditation after it had been achieved because the study time frame did not allow observation of MMT for an appropriate follow-up period to ascertain such costs.

SUMMARY

- The Evaluation Study was a nationally representative study of MMT programs in the late 1990s.

- The focus of this book is on descriptive analyses of 172 MMT programs' data collected during a preaccreditation visit.

- The Evaluation Study collected data at the program, staff, and patient levels.

CHAPTER 4—Methadone Maintenance Treatment Program Characteristics

How programs approach daily MMT is often shaped by organizational characteristics, including the number of patients they serve, their ownership, their location, how long they have been in operation, and their stability. This chapter examines these characteristics along with key practices such as patient assessment, quality assurance, treatment orientation, emergency access, and community input.

HOW MANY PATIENTS DO MMT PROGRAMS SERVE?

The number of patients MMT programs serve is an important factor in shaping and reflecting resource needs and the treatment experience. The size of MMT programs has been increasing over time. In 1987, for example, the average daily census was 129 patients; by 1992, it had increased to 182 patients (D'Aunno & Vaughn, 1992).

MMT program size, by patient census, is shown in Figure 4.1. The mean program size was 253 patients; the smallest program in the study had 20 patients, and the largest had just under 2,000. About 20% of the programs had fewer than 100 patients, and about 32% had more than 300.

Figure 4.1 MMT Program Size, by Patient Census

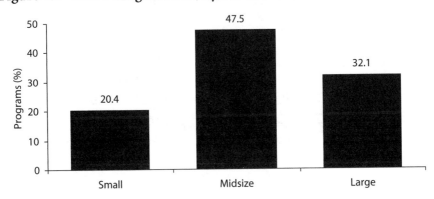

Note: Small = 0–100 patients; midsize = 101–300 patients; large = 301 or more patients.

WHO OWNS MMT PROGRAMS?

Ownership of MMT programs has long been considered an important factor affecting services. For example, Wheeler and Nahra (2000) found that patients in for-profit substance abuse treatment programs differed substantially from patients at nonprofit or public programs, suggesting the emergence of a two-tiered system of care. Wheeler, Fadel, and D'Aunno (1992) found significant differences in patients, services, access to services, and expenditures across ownership models. McCaughrin and Price (1992) found better outcomes in for-profit programs.

The number of for-profit MMT programs has been increasing in recent years. In 1997, less than one-third of MMT programs (30%) were for-profit organizations. By 2004, that number had increased to nearly half (48%).

Approximately 46% of the programs in the study were for-profit organizations; the remaining 54% were nonprofit or government owned. About 70% of the MMT programs in the study were part of a larger entity (i.e., had a parent organization); 30% were single-site programs. MMT programs owned by a single parent organization may operate under universal administrative policies and fiscal management.

WHERE ARE MMT PROGRAMS LOCATED?

MMT programs originated in large urban areas, such as New York City. Big cities still house the majority of MMT programs; however, recent decades have seen more programs operating in smaller cities, suburbs, exurbs, and rural areas. Policy makers are particularly concerned about access to MMT in rural areas.

MMT programs in the study were predominantly located in urban or large urban areas (Figure 4.2). About two-thirds of the programs (67%) were located in large urban areas with a county population greater than 1 million. A quarter (25%) of the programs were located in urban areas with a county population between 250,000 and 1 million; the remaining 8% of programs were located in nonurban areas (i.e., counties) with a population of less than 250,000.

Figure 4.2 Proportion of MMT Programs, by Urbanicity

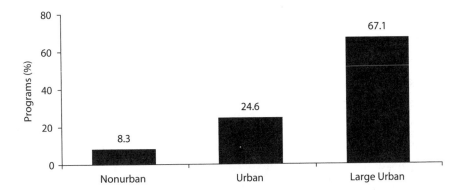

Note: Nonurban = county population < 250,000; urban = county population 250,000–1,000,000; large urban = county population > 1,000,000.

HOW LONG HAVE MMT PROGRAMS BEEN OPERATING?

On average, MMT programs in the study had been providing treatment services for 16 years. The oldest program had been in operation for more than 30 years, and the newest program had been in operation for less than 1 year.

Much of the recent growth in the methadone treatment system has been in the for-profit sector. On average, for-profit programs were founded more recently than nonprofit or government-operated programs. Over half of the for-profit programs (53%) had been in operation for 10 years or less, compared with 30% of nonprofit programs.

HOW STABLE ARE MMT PROGRAMS?

MMT programs operate in turbulent environments, facing shifting demands and changes both internally and externally (in funding, oversight, and treatment options). The Services Research Outcomes Study (SROS) found that 20% of MMT programs in the sample had new ownership or administration between 1990 and 1994 (OAS, 1998). The average annual staff turnover rate was about 20%. In a review of findings on methadone treatment, Farrell et al. (1994) concluded that organizational stability, as evidenced by sound clinic management and low staff turnover rates, was

linked to better treatment outcomes. Ball and Ross (1991) found organizational stability to be one factor in treatment effectiveness. In related work,
Magura, Nwakeze, Kang, and Demsky (1999) found an association between
treatment effectiveness and site director involvement and experience.

The MMT programs in the Evaluation Study were experiencing a fair
amount of organizational change. In the 6 months preceding the baseline site
visit, approximately 40% had undergone a major change, such as new ownership, a new site director, or new approaches to treatment. Almost 20% of the
programs had experienced one such event, close to 16% had experienced
two events, and nearly 6% had experienced all three events in the 6 months
before baseline data collection. About 18% reported extensive staff turnover
in the 6 months before data collection.

In written responses to an open-ended question about other changes
their programs had experienced in the previous 6 months, 12 clinical directors identified some aspect of growth or expansion (e.g., growth of clinic,
expanded HIV services) and 11 identified staffing issues (including staff
illnesses or deaths, as well as staff changes, such as contracts with pharmacists). Other changes mentioned included facility issues, such as a new facility
or extensive repairs (mentioned by two respondents); oversight issues,
including new state certification and investigations (mentioned by three
respondents); and financial issues (mentioned by two respondents). Three
respondents noted accreditation issues as other major events in the previous
6 months.

HOW DO MMT PROGRAMS ASSESS AND EVALUATE PATIENT NEEDS?

MMT programs are required by federal regulations to assess each patient
at intake and reassess patients periodically to ensure that adequate services
are available as needed. The initial assessment must include a treatment plan;
requirements for education, vocational rehabilitation, and employment; and
needs for medical, psychosocial, economic, legal, and other support
services.

A wide variety of instruments are used to screen for patient substance
abuse problems. Many of the most popular screening instruments (e.g., the

Michigan Alcoholism Screening Test [MAST]; Cut Down, Annoyed, Guilty, Eye Opener [CAGE]; Alcohol Use Disorders Identification Test [AUDIT]) were either designed for alcohol use or are more sensitive to problems associated with alcohol use and are therefore less appropriate for use in MMT programs. Other screening tools (e.g., the Drug Abuse Screening Test [DAST], Substance Abuse Subtle Screening Inventory [SASSI]) are more appropriate for use in substance-abusing populations. These instruments have been found to be sensitive and reliable indicators of substance abuse problems.

Screening instruments do not typically provide detailed diagnoses of alcohol and other drug use problems, and they do not provide reliable benchmarks for assessing whether patients are progressing in their treatment. For this reason, patient progress is usually monitored using a combination of medical tests (e.g., drug testing), clinical interviewing, and assessment instruments.

The Addiction Severity Index (ASI) is considered to be a versatile assessment tool (McLellan et al., 1992). It has been used since 1980 and has been modified extensively over the years to account for trends in substance abuse. The ASI is a semistructured instrument that can be used to measure the overall severity of addiction and can follow a respondent's progress while in treatment. The questions are grouped into seven functional areas: (1) medical status, (2) employment, (3) drug use, (4) alcohol use, (5) legal status, (6) family/social status, and (7) psychiatric status. The instrument focuses on the frequency of problems, their duration, and their lifetime and past-month severity. Answers are scored on a scale of 0 (not at all) to 5 (extreme), which reflects the need for treatment in that area. For each of the seven areas, the test administrator rates the respondent's degree of need on a scale of 1 to 10. Scores for each of the areas are summed; the higher the scores, the greater the need for treatment.

The ASI has several advantages over other screening instruments. First, it is in the public domain and is therefore free to administer. Second, the amount of training required to administer it is small compared with training for more elaborate assessment tools. Because the ASI has been used for over 20 years, it has been found to be valid and reliable in both research and clinical settings. Unlike briefer screening instruments, the ASI can be used to track patients' progress during treatment. The ASI has also been shown to be valid across a wide variety of treatment modalities (e.g., inpatient and outpatient), populations (e.g., heroin and cocaine users), and languages (e.g., Spanish and French editions).

To examine how MMT programs conduct patient treatment assessments, the Evaluation Study asked clinical directors and other staff members in each of the programs about assessment processes, assessment instruments used, use of placement criteria, and frequency of periodic reassessments. The results indicated the following:

- Virtually all of the treatment programs assessed patients in numerous areas, including substance use and abuse history, psychiatric health, social environment and family, education and work, physical health, and criminal background.

- More than half of all MMT programs (56%) required staff to use specific placement criteria when placing all patients; use of these criteria was required for only some patients in 7% of the programs and for no patients in 37% of the programs.

- Although 76% of the programs used *Diagnostic and Statistical Manual of Mental Disorders* (DSM-IV) criteria and 66% used their own criteria to assess patients, there was notable variation across programs in the mix of criteria used: almost 21% of the programs used DSM-IV and program-specific criteria, and almost 16% used DSM-IV, American Society of Addiction Medicine (ASAM), and program-specific criteria (Figure 4.3).

- The majority of MMT program staff reported that they relied mainly on a program-specific patient assessment instrument (Figure 4.4). Approximately 7% of staff reported using the ASI along with a program-specific instrument, and 5% of staff reported using no assessment instrument. About 30% of staff reported using a variety of instruments. The most commonly used standardized instrument was the ASI.

• Nearly 46% of the program staff conducted patient assessments more frequently than annually, and about 36% of the staff conducted them as needed (Figure 4.5). Half used the same instrument or protocol used at intake for reassessment of patient needs.

The variation in assessment procedures and practices indicates that MMT programs lacked a consistent patient assessment process at the time of the study.

Figure 4.3   Patient Assessment Criteria Used in MMT Programs

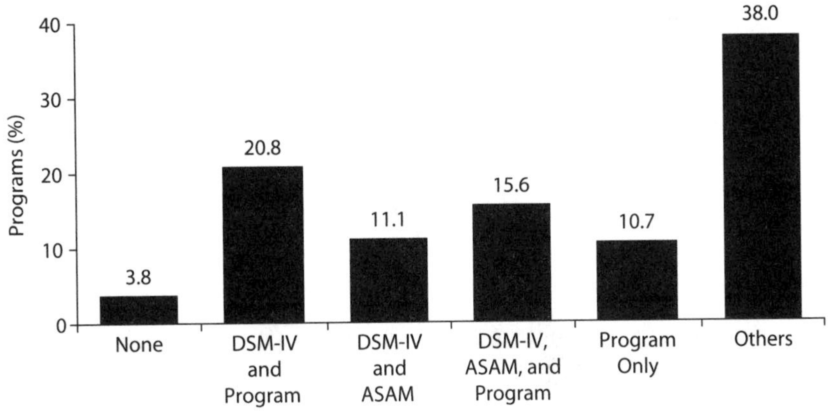

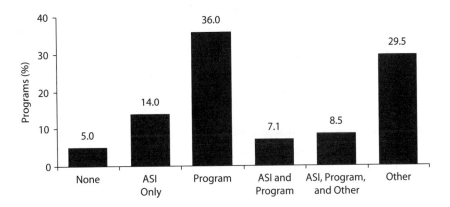

Figure 4.4   Patient Assessment Instruments Used in MTT Programs

Note: Because of rounding, percentages do not sum to exactly 100.

Figure 4.5   Frequency of Patient Assessments in MMT Programs

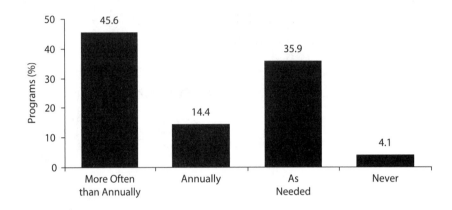

WHAT QUALITY ASSURANCE ACTIVITIES ARE USED TO ASSESS PERFORMANCE?

The 1990 GAO report on MMT indicated that very few MMT programs used quality assurance (QA) methods to assess their own performance and effectiveness (GAO, 1990).

To understand the structure and scope of QA policies at MMT programs, the study asked clinical directors about their QA processes. The findings showed that almost all MMT programs (95%) reported having an ongoing QA procedure in place, and 84% reported having written QA procedures.

To better understand which activities were included in MMT programs' QA systems, the study asked clinical directors about specific activities undertaken as part of standard procedures. Figure 4.6 shows the percentage of MMT programs reporting each of the activities. Nearly 96% of programs reported holding regular QA meetings, and nearly 99% reported reviewing patient charts for completeness. Although federal regulations strongly emphasize outcome monitoring, only about 69% of programs reported monitoring trends and collecting data on outcome indicators.

To help assess the resources that MMT programs committed to QA, the study asked clinical directors whether their programs had a QA staff position. Overall, only 46% of all programs reported having a staff member dedicated to QA either part-time or full-time. Additionally, clinical directors reported that their programs used verbal information from staff (92%), written information prepared specifically for a QA meeting (79%), or patient charts (82%) as sources of information for QA rather than information obtained from a program database (69%).

Figure 4.6 Quality Assurance Activities in MMT Programs

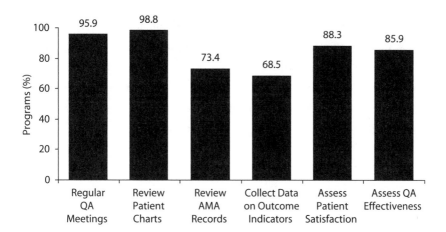

Note: Because multiple responses were allowed, percentages do not sum to 100.

DO MMT PROGRAMS DIFFER IN THEIR TREATMENT ORIENTATION?

Studies have examined MMT orientation in a variety of ways. The early Drug Abuse Reporting Program (DARP) classification of programs by treatment orientation yielded two models: adaptive and change oriented (Sells & Simpson, 1976). Adaptive programs were those that offered a supportive therapeutic method, placed few demands on patients, accepted that ongoing drug use occurred, strived to reduce crises, and expected ongoing treatment or maintenance. Change-oriented programs offered highly structured treatment, defined expectations for patient behavior, aimed to resocialize patients, and expected that treatment would be time limited (e.g., Joe et al., 1983).

A later classification categorized programs as reformist or libertarian. Reformist programs offered only low doses of methadone, limited patients' time in treatment, and decreased doses following positive urinalysis results.

Libertarian programs offered higher doses, did not limit time in treatment, and increased doses following positive urinalysis results (Caplehorn, McNeil, & Kleinbaum, 1993).

A more recent variation classified methadone programs as reformist, medical model, and libertarian (Kelley, 2001). Reformist programs exercised the most control over patients, whereas libertarian programs offered the most laissez-faire approach to treatment. Kelley found the greatest treatment effectiveness in the medical-model programs, which acknowledged the challenging, shifting nature of addiction and permitted patients to make choices in their treatment.

Using this idea of treatment orientation, three descriptive measures were developed for the Evaluation Study. The first measure assessed treatment **philosophy** and was defined by the following characteristics:

- implementation of dosage caps
- implementation of time limits on treatment
- maximum methadone dose
- encouragement of detoxification
- encouragement of participation in Alcoholics Anonymous and Narcotics Anonymous as part of treatment
- likelihood of verbal reprimands for two consecutive positive tests

Programs at the low end of the philosophy score distribution were patient centered and maintenance oriented, as indicated by the following characteristics:

- no dosage cap
- no time limit on treatment
- 1,100 mg maximum dose
- some encouragement of detoxification
- some encouragement of participation in Alcoholics Anonymous and Narcotics Anonymous

- verbal reprimands extremely unlikely for two consecutive positive urine tests

Programs at the high end of the philosophy score distribution were program centered and rehabilitation oriented, as indicated by the following characteristics:

- dosage cap

- time limit on treatment

- 50 mg maximum dose

- great encouragement of detoxification

- great encouragement of participation in Alcoholics Anonymous and Narcotics Anonymous

- verbal reprimands extremely likely for two consecutive positive urine tests

The second measure focused on **practice** in the realm of clarity of expectations and program consequences for continued illicit opioid use. It was defined by the following characteristics:

- likelihood of loss of privileges for two consecutive positive urine tests

- likelihood of revision of treatment plans for two consecutive positive urine tests

- likelihood of discharge for two consecutive positive urine tests

Programs at the low end of the practice distribution score had a laissez-faire approach, as indicated by the following characteristics:

- loss of privileges unlikely for two consecutive positive urine tests

- revision of treatment plans unlikely for two consecutive positive urine tests

- discharge extremely unlikely for two consecutive positive urine tests

At the high end of the practice distribution score were programs with a clear consequences approach, as indicated by the following characteristics:

- loss of privileges extremely likely for two consecutive positive urine tests
- revision of treatment plans extremely likely for two consecutive positive urine tests
- discharge likely for two consecutive positive urine tests

The third measure assessed **patient involvement in dosing** and was defined by the following characteristics:

- extent to which patients were informed when their dosage changed
- extent to which patients influenced decisions about dosage

The high and low ends of the distribution score for this measure were as follows. At the low end, patients were sometimes informed when their dosage changed, and patients influenced their dosage to some extent. At the high end, patients were always informed when their dosage changed, and patients influenced their dosage to a great extent.

Evaluators examined associations between the treatment orientation variables and the three organizational characteristics of size, ownership, and location. No association was found between these variables and ownership or location. Treatment orientation, as defined here, does not appear to vary according to ownership or urbanicity. There was no association between size and treatment practice or patient involvement in dosing. However, evaluators did find a statistically significant association between size and the treatment philosophy measure. The largest sites had the lowest scores, indicating that they were more likely to offer maintenance-oriented treatment, with higher doses and no time limit on treatment.

HOW DO MMT PROGRAMS PROVIDE SERVICES DURING AN EMERGENCY OR DISASTER?

Federal regulations call for MMT programs to have designated staff available 24 hours a day, 7 days a week. Programs can meet this requirement in several ways; for example, they can have staff on call or arrange for a 24-hour crisis line to provide after-hours coverage.

Findings from the study show that about 84% of MMT programs provided at least one method of responding to after-hours patient emergencies, as shown in Figure 4.7. At nearly 56% of the programs, patients were given a 24-hour emergency service telephone number to contact a community crisis intervention agency for after-hours emergencies. Nearly 44% of the programs provided pagers or cellular phones for the program staff to respond to emergencies, and nearly 21% of the programs employed 24-hour emergency workers. About 10% of the programs used other means, including voice mail, hospital emergency rooms for medical services, a 24-hour nursing service, and answering machines with emergency instructions.

Figure 4.7   MMT Program Policies for Ensuring 24-Hour Access to Emergency Care

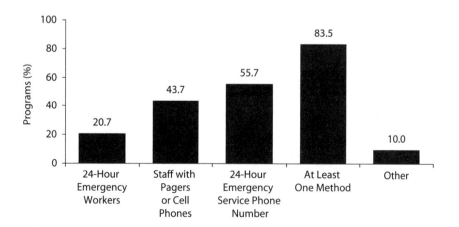

Note: Because multiple responses were allowed, percentages do not sum to 100.

DO MMT PROGRAMS SEEK INPUT FROM THEIR COMMUNITIES?

Accreditation standards call for community input on MMT program impact. Programs can obtain community input in a variety of ways. For example, 85% of MMT programs in the study (146 of 172) had a governing board. Of the 146 programs with a governing board, 64% included community representation. Nonprofit or public programs were more likely to include community representation on their board: nearly 90% of nonprofit/public programs with a governing board included community representation, compared with about one-quarter (26%) of for-profit programs.

SUMMARY

- The majority of MMT programs in the Evaluation Study were part of a larger organizational entity.

- The majority of MMT programs operated in larger urban settings.

- Almost all MMT programs had QA measures in place, which typically included reviewing patient charts and holding regular QA meetings; however, less than a third of the programs collected outcome indicators.

- MMT treatment orientation can be characterized along three dimensions: treatment philosophy, treatment practice, and patient involvement in dosing. The findings suggest great variability across programs.

- Over a third of MMT programs reported requiring no specific criteria when placing patients in treatment.

- The largest MMT programs in the study had the lowest treatment orientation scores, indicating that they were more likely to offer maintenance-oriented treatment, with higher doses and no time limit on treatment.

CHAPTER 5—Core and Ancillary Methadone Maintenance Treatment Services

This chapter reviews the broad range of core services (counseling and treatment) and ancillary services (e.g., educational, vocational) provided in MMT. We examine differences by ownership, size, and location, as covered in the Evaluation Study, and conclude with a discussion of special services provided to vulnerable populations.

WHAT SERVICES DO MMT PROGRAMS PROVIDE?

Many patients come to MMT programs with concurrent physical and psychological problems. Although medication services alone may be sufficient to produce positive outcomes for some patients, for others this is not the case. Federal regulations require MMT programs to provide adequate medical, counseling, vocational, educational, and other assessment and treatment services for patients who need them.

Patient services are categorized into two groups: core and ancillary. Core services include medical care (general medical and AIDS-related medical care), psychological services, and treatment for drugs other than heroin (detoxification from a substance other than heroin; treatment for addiction to alcohol, cocaine, or other illicit drugs). Ancillary services include educational, vocational, financial, legal, family, housing/shelter, acupuncture, transportation, and child care services.

Studies have shown that the availability of services other than methadone dosing, such as counseling and psychological services, is associated with lower relapse rates and greater retention in treatment (Joe et al., 1991; McLellan et al., 1993). In particular, counseling services have been found to be related to positive treatment outcomes. Ball and Ross (1991), in a study replicated by Magura et al. (1999), found that a greater frequency of counseling contacts was positively associated with treatment outcomes. McLellan et al. found that patients with regular, supervised counseling showed greater

improvements more quickly than patients receiving methadone dosing and
no other services. From the evidence gathered in studies of the effectiveness
of core and ancillary services, the IOM recommended that regulations
support patients' access to a comprehensive array of services (Rettig &
Yarmolinsky, 1995).

The Evaluation Study found that most MMT patients received individual
counseling services at the program site: about 88% of programs reported
providing individual counseling to virtually all of their patients (81% to
100%; Figure 5.1). Group counseling was much less common. Almost half of
the programs reported providing on-site group counseling to 10% or less of
their patients, and just over 20% provided group counseling to more than
60% of their patients.

Figure 5.1 Individual and Group MMT Counseling Services

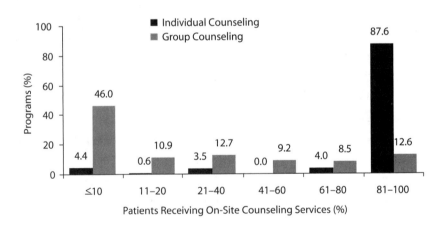

Nearly all MMT programs reported offering core services: 93% offered
general medical services, 97% offered AIDS-related services, 98% offered
psychological services, 93% provided detoxification from a substance other
than heroin, 97% offered treatment for alcohol dependence, 95% offered
treatment for cocaine dependence, and 96% offered treatment for addiction
to other illicit drugs.

WHAT SERVICES DO MMT PATIENTS REPORT RECEIVING?

Program directors were asked to report the average number of times per month patients received both individual and group counseling services at the program site. Based on the information provided by program directors, the mean number of times per month patients received individual or group counseling sessions on-site was nearly equal. Patients received an average of 2.4 individual counseling sessions per month and an average of 2.8 group counseling sessions.

When asked specifically about treatment services received during the 3 months before the survey, most MMT patients reported receiving individual counseling (78%), which they received more than any other service (Figure 5.2). The services reported as received least during the previous 3 months were legal assistance (8%) and housing/shelter assistance (7%). Although these low percentages partially reflect limitations in service availability, they also reflect the lack of ongoing need for these services for many patients in MMT.

Figure 5.2 Services Received by MMT Patients

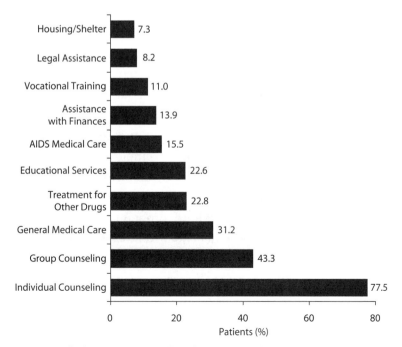

Note: Because multiple responses were allowed, percentages do not sum to 100.

HOW DO MMT PROGRAMS PROVIDE CORE AND ANCILLARY SERVICES?

The location and delivery of ancillary and treatment-related services has been found to be associated with the likelihood that patients receive these services. Centralized delivery may lower barriers to services, such as the cost to patients, transportation problems, lifestyle disorganization, and stigma (Friedmann, Lemon, Stein, Etheridge, & D'Aunno, 2001). A random trial of 51 hospital-based methadone patients in Baltimore found that those who were offered medical care on-site were more likely to obtain it than those offered care at a medical clinic on the same campus (Umbricht-Schneiter, Ginn, Pabst, & Bigelow, 1994). On-site availability of primary care services may be particularly important to methadone patients who are HIV-positive. One study found that this group was more likely to use services and that frequency of visits increased as a function of declining CD4 counts (Selwyn, Budner, Wasserman, & Arno, 1993).

Programs vary greatly in whether they provide treatment services directly (i.e., at the program location) or through other arrangements (e.g., through referrals to other programs or other community service organizations). How core and ancillary services are delivered (i.e., on-site versus at another of the MMT's program's sites or through referral) is associated with how likely patients are to receive these services. On-site delivery may lower barriers to services, such as the cost to patients, transportation problems, lifestyle disorganization, and stigma. Exclusive on-site delivery of medical services in the first month of treatment has been found to be related to increased utilization of medical services, compared with informal referral only. Delivery of on-site medical, psychological, employment, and financial counseling services at outpatient drug treatment and MMT facilities has also been associated with greater patient service utilization.

The Evaluation Study examined how programs provided specific services, such as treatment for drug dependence other than heroin (Table 5.1) and medical and psychological services (Table 5.2). MMT programs provided treatment for abuse of alcohol, cocaine, or other drugs similarly. Approximately half offered treatment on-site or through formal links with other programs, fewer offered the service at another of their program's locations, and most also offered services for other drug dependence through informal links with other programs.

Table 5.1   Provision of Treatment for Other Drug Dependence

	On-site	At Other Program Sites/Not On-site	Offered (%) Through Formal Links Only	Through Informal Links Only	Treatment Not Provided
Treatment for Other Drug Dependence					
Alcohol	52.1	31.0	48.4	84.9	3.2
Cocaine	55.6	25.0	47.2	82.2	4.5
Other Drugs	53.5	24.7	45.7	83.6	3.9

Note: Because multiple responses were allowed, percentages sum to greater than 100.

Table 5.2   Provision of Treatment for Medical and Psychological Services

	On-site	At Other Program Sites/Not On-site	Offered (%) Through Formal Links Only	Through Informal Links Only	Treatment Not Provided
Treatment for Other Drug Dependence					
General Medical Care	37.4	22.2	46.7	83.0	6.5
AIDS-Related Care	22.0	21.8	51.4	84.6	2.5
Psychological Services	45.4	28.0	53.6	85.0	2.0

Note: Because multiple responses were allowed, percentages sum to greater than 100.

About half of the programs provided general medical care or AIDS-related care on-site or through another location of their program; access to this type of care was most commonly offered through linkages with other organizations. Psychological services were more likely to be offered on-site or at other locations of the same program. The arrangements that programs used to provide general medical care, AIDS-related care, and psychological services were generally predictive of how they offered other medical and psychological services.

Evaluation research analysts examined program service delivery systems by defining mutually exclusive categories for delivery (Berkman & Wechsberg, in press). When defined as mutually exclusive categories, 40% of programs reported offering general medical care on-site, and 22% of programs offered AIDS-related medical care on-site. By far, the majority of services for both general medical care and AIDS-related care were offered by programs through formal (27% and 38%, respectively) or informal (25% and 28%, respectively) links.

Although most programs offered transportation assistance (62%) and child care (71%), less than half offered either of these services directly. In more than half of the programs, assistance in obtaining child care was provided only through indirect arrangements (giving patients information or referring them to other organizations; Figure 5.3). The arrangement used to provide transportation services was significantly related to the arrangement used for providing child care. That is, programs that provided transportation services on-site, such as through vouchers or staff pickup, were significantly more likely to also provide child care services on-site or provide financial assistance for obtaining care elsewhere.

Although most MMT programs reported providing access to ancillary services, these services were not commonly provided on-site or at another program location. Only one-quarter of the programs provided vocational services—the most commonly provided ancillary service—on-site or at another program location. Access to these and other ancillary services was most likely to be offered through informal links to other programs (Table 5.3). The arrangements that programs used to provide educational, vocational, financial, legal, and housing/shelter services were all significantly related, meaning that programs tended to provide each of the services through similar arrangements.

Evaluation research analysts also examined ancillary program service delivery systems by defining mutually exclusive categories for delivery (Berkman & Wechsberg, in press). When defined as mutually exclusive categories, only 12% of programs reported providing educational assistance on-site; 21% reported providing vocational services on-site; 14% reported providing financial assistance on-site; 4% reported providing legal assistance; and 9% reported providing assistance with housing on-site. The majority of programs reported providing ancillary services through informal links. Additionally, over 20% of programs reported not providing financial or legal assistance at all (21% and 22%, respectively).

Figure 5.3 Provision of Transportation and Child Care Services

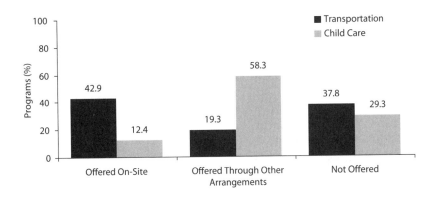

Table 5.3 Provision of Other Ancillary Services

	Offered (%)				
	On-site	**At Other Program Sites/Not On-site**	**Through Formal Links Only**	**Through Informal Links Only**	**Treatment Not Provided**
Ancillary Service					
Educational	13.8	13.9	34.6	84.0	8.3
Vocational	19.4	14.5	41.5	84.1	5.4
Financial	9.5	5.7	16.4	72.7	23.1
Legal	2.3	2.4	15.5	77.5	20.0
Housing/ Shelter	6.7	6.8	27.6	91.3	5.6

Note: Because multiple responses were allowed, percentages sum to greater than 100.

Generally, few MMT programs offered both core and ancillary services on-site. Programs seemed to adhere to one type of service delivery arrangement (e.g., services offered through referral) for all types of treatment services. The lack of on-site services provided to MMT patients is troubling in light of the evidence supporting the treatment and recovery benefits associated with on-site care.

HOW DOES SERVICE DELIVERY DIFFER BY ORGANIZATIONAL OWNERSHIP AND SIZE?

The Evaluation Study examined the availability of services in relation to two variables important in developing regulation policy: ownership type (e.g., for-profit and nonprofit [including government]) and number of patients (size of a program).

Educational services were more likely to be provided by programs on-site or through another program location at nonprofit programs, compared with for-profit programs (27% versus 16%). For-profit programs were more likely to offer educational services through informal links, compared with nonprofit programs (69% versus 31%; Table 5.4).

The study found similar results for program delivery of other ancillary services. For example, 22% of nonprofit programs reported providing vocational services on-site, compared with only 6% of for-profit programs. Again, for-profit programs reported primarily providing vocational services through informal links (60%, compared with only 28% of nonprofit programs).

Large programs reported the highest percentage for offering financial services on-site to patients (16%, compared with 11% for small programs and 3% for midsize programs). Small, midsize, and large programs reported offering the majority of their patients financial services through informal links in the community (45%, 63%, and 52%, respectively). No significant relationship was found between the delivery of educational, vocational, or housing services and program size.

Table 5.4   Provision of Other Ancillary Services, by Ownership

		Offered (%)			
	On-site	At Other Program Sites/Not On-site	Through Formal Links Only	Through Informal Links Only	Service Not Provided
Educational					
For-profit	14.1	2.3	12.8	68.9	2.1
Nonprofit/public	9.8	17.1	31.9	31.3	10.2
Vocational					
For-profit	6.6	0.0	26.6	60.3	6.6
Nonprofit/public	22.1	13.1	31.4	28.4	5.0
Housing/Shelter					
For-profit	2.2	0.0	11.6	81.9	4.3
Nonprofit/public	4.8	11.3	35.8	44.7	3.5

Note: Because multiple responses were allowed, percentages sum to greater than 100.

WHAT SPECIALIZED SERVICES DO MMT PROGRAMS PROVIDE TO VULNERABLE POPULATIONS?

Figure 5.4 shows the distribution of specialized services for vulnerable populations. More than half of the MMT programs offered specialized services on-site for women, pregnant women, and patients with HIV/AIDS. Generally, programs providing specialized services for one of the groups in Figure 5.4 were significantly more likely to provide specialized services for the other groups presented in the figure. The exception is provision of specialized services for patients involved with the criminal justice system, which was rare.

Nonprofit programs were significantly more likely than for-profit programs to provide specialized services for females, patients with HIV/AIDS, and patients with psychiatric diagnoses. No significant differences by ownership type were found in the provision of services for non-English-speaking patients, pregnant women, or patients with involvement in the criminal justice system (Figure 5.5).

Figure 5.4   Distribution of Specialized Services for Vulnerable Populations

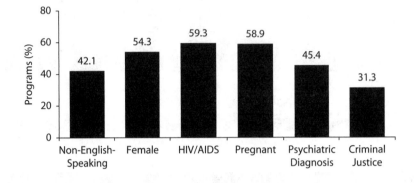

Note: Because multiple responses were allowed, percentages sum to greater than 100.

Figure 5.5   Provision of Specialized Services for Vulnerable Populations, by Ownership

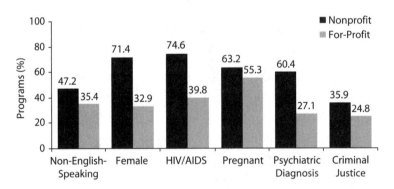

Note: Because multiple responses were allowed, percentages sum to greater than 100.

Specialized services for women were more likely to be provided at larger programs, and specialized services for pregnant women were more likely to be provided at midsize programs. About 72% of midsize programs, compared with 39% of small programs and 51% of large programs, offered specialized services for pregnant women. Program size was not associated with other specialized services for vulnerable populations.

SUMMARY

- Most MMT programs offered individual counseling to virtually all of their patients, as well as a variety of other core services.

- Many core and ancillary services were most often offered informally to patients, which could have a negative effect on whether the services were received.

- In the previous 3 months, patients were most likely to report receiving individual counseling (78%), group counseling (43%), and general medical care (31%); they were least likely to report receiving legal (8%) and housing/shelter assistance (7%).

- Nonprofit programs were more likely than for-profit programs to offer educational services and transportation services.

- Nonprofit programs offered more comprehensive services on-site or through links than for-profit programs.

- Not all programs provided specialized services, but nonprofits offered many more services to vulnerable populations, compared with for-profit programs. The populations served included women, patients living with HIV/AIDS, and patients diagnosed with a psychiatric disorder.

CHAPTER 6—Dosing Practices in Methadone Maintenance Treatment Programs

Practices vary widely in methadone dosing, the core service of MMT programs. In this chapter, we review the various approaches to methadone administration. We present average dosing levels, discuss physician practices for determining dosing levels, and explore take-home medication practices. The chapter concludes with a discussion of methadone diversion and methadone-related mortality.

WHAT ARE THE PRINCIPAL APPROACHES TO METHADONE DOSING?

Seivewright (2000) identified two main approaches that MMT programs commonly take. The first approach, long-term MMT, uses methadone as a medication to correct a disorder and tends to provide treatment for an indefinite period. The second approach, abstinence-oriented treatment, seeks to provide methadone for a limited time and urges withdrawal. These two approaches, known as the *medical model* and the *substitution model*, respectively, are based on different rationales for treatment and use methadone dosing differently (Seivewright, 2000).

The data presented in this book come from some MMT programs implementing the medical model of opiate dependence treatment and others implementing an abstinence-oriented model. In the medical model, methadone dosing is used as a means to correct the metabolic disturbance caused by opiate dependence (Dole & Nyswander, 1965). By reducing craving and blocking the effects of other opiates, methadone improves patients' physical and psychological health when they are given an adequate dosage for an indefinite period. Therefore, the value of maintenance treatment lies primarily in the opportunity it provides for dependent drug users to reduce their exposure to risk behaviors and stabilize their health and social situations.

In the medical model, patients are initially prescribed a lower dosage of methadone (e.g., 30 mg); the daily dose is then increased to an adequate level to suppress craving and effectively block the effects of other opiates. In their seminal study of six methadone treatment programs, Ball and Ross (1991) recommended that maintenance dosages of at least 80 mg a day be prescribed on a long-term basis without having patients reduce their dosages or withdraw from methadone.

HOW IS METHADONE ADMINISTERED?

Methadone is the most widely applied and researched medication for opiate dependence agonist pharmacotherapy. Some emerging medications, including buprenorphine, work similarly and are an important addition to the field of opiate dependence treatment, but it is beyond the scope of this book to discuss them in detail.

Methadone is usually administered orally as a liquid in a single daily dose, which is prescribed to prevent withdrawal symptoms for 24 hours. Oral methadone, whether used for addiction treatment or pain relief, is available as a solid tablet, a rapidly dissolving wafer (diskette), and a premixed liquid, all of which are essentially bioequivalent (Mallinckrodt, 1995, 2000). Under FDA regulations, MMT programs were restricted to the use of liquid methadone. The Final Rule eliminated these restrictions (DHHS, 2001).

WHAT DOSING LEVELS ARE USED IN MMT?

The approach to treating opiate dependence has changed since methadone was first used as an agonist pharmacotherapy. MMT has been provided according to different models and in keeping with multitiered regulations and policies. According to Seivewright (2000), the United States has favored the use of lower dosages of methadone (e.g., 60 mg) in MMT, in part because of a low acceptance of long-term maintenance. Financial and political factors based on ideological beliefs, which include low acceptance of opiate dependence as a medical disorder requiring long-term treatment, have played a significant role in supporting the acceptance of these practices (Rosenbaum, 1995). Following the emergence of the HIV/AIDS epidemic and the discovery of its link to injection drug use, however, attention was refocused on providing effective treatment with higher dosages of methadone for IDUs. The relationship between HIV/AIDS and opiate use, coupled with the demonstrated effectiveness of MMT in reducing the spread of HIV/AIDS, added impetus to maintaining dependent persons on higher levels of methadone (Cooper, 1989).

CSAT's state methadone treatment guidelines recommend that an effective dosage is likely to be about 80 mg a day, plus or minus 20 mg (Parrino, 1993). IOM recommended that dosing restrictions other than the initial 30-mg dose be removed from methadone regulations (Rettig & Yarmolinsky, 1995). CSAT guidelines concur with the IOM recommendations, with the intent of providing physicians with a greater margin for professional discretion in prescribing and adjusting maintenance dosages. The Final Rule created latitude for physicians by removing the FDA regulation requiring federal approval for dosages over 100 mg a day (DHHS, 2001a).

WHAT RESTRICTIONS ARE PLACED ON INITIAL METHADONE DOSING?

CSAT (2001) emphasized the importance of providing physicians with broad latitude to exercise clinical judgment in initial dosing; the current federal regulation is 30 to 40 mg at admission. If this dose is exceeded, the rationale should be documented in the patient's chart. The CSAT accreditation guidelines and individual accreditation organization standards are in agreement with this regulation.

As part of the Evaluation Study, MMT program directors were queried about the typical admission dosage prescribed at their programs. The findings show that the average admission dosage at MMT programs was about 34 mg a day. This mean dosage is within the recommended guidelines; it is over 30 mg but under 40 mg. The overall range of reported admission dosages was 15 to 80 mg.

WHAT IS THE AVERAGE MMT DOSAGE?

Methadone dosages of 60 to 100 mg a day or more have been identified as being most effective in retaining patients in treatment and reducing illicit drug use and criminal behavior (Kreek, 2000; Parrino, 1993; Ward, Mattick, & Hall, 1998). Debate continues, however, over what constitutes an appropriate average daily dose.

According to Payte (1997), MMT programs tend to prescribe low dosages. Payte posits that this tendency is a function of regulations focused on abstinence rather than on rehabilitation. Researchers and MMT staff have recognized that suboptimal dosing contributes to the continued use of opiates. Randomized clinical trial results (Ling, Wesson, Charuvastra, & Klett, 1996; Schottenfeld, Pakes, Oliveto, Ziedonis, & Kosten, 1997; Strain, Stitzer, Liebson, & Bigelow, 1993) and retrospective outcomes analyses of clinical populations (Caplehorn & Bell, 1991; Maremmani, Nardini, Zolesi, & Castrogiovanni, 1994) have shown that higher dosages of methadone are associated with lower rates of opiate and other drug use, as well as increased retention in treatment. Temporary increases in dosages have also been found to decrease illicit drug use and improve social functioning (Gossup, Strang, & Connell, 1982). Moreover, Dole (1988), Metzger and Platt (1987), and Strain, Bigelow, Liebson, and Stitzer (1999) demonstrated that dosages higher than 80 mg a day are effective and safe.

Research results demonstrate that, contrary to Payte's (1997) contention of low dosing, there has been a consistent increase in the average maintenance dosage from 1988 through 2000. D'Aunno and Vaughn (1992) reported that the average maintenance dosage of methadone among 172 treatment facilities was 45 mg a day in 1988. In 1995, D'Aunno and Vaughn (1995) reported that the average dosage at 140 MMT programs was 59 mg a day, with an average upper limit of 93 mg a day—a considerable increase over the 1990 level of 82 mg. In the most recent review of dosing levels, D'Aunno and Pollack (2002) indicated that the percentage of patients receiving less than the recommended 60 mg a day had decreased from 79.5% in 1988 to 35.5% in 2000.

To gather information about dosing practices at MMT programs, the Evaluation Study analyzed the percentage of patients receiving maintenance dosages within particular ranges, the average maintenance dosage, and the largest dosage currently prescribed across programs, by program ownership status, size, and program location (e.g., urban versus rural).

The study asked program directors to list the proportion of patients in treatment for at least 2 weeks who received maintenance dosages within the following categories: less than 40 mg a day, 40 to 59 mg a day, 60 to 79 mg a day, 80 to 99 mg a day, and 100 mg a day or more. Figure 6.1 shows the mean proportion of patients receiving dosages in each of these categories.

Figure 6.1   Patients in Treatment at Least 2 Weeks Receiving Methadone Maintenance Doses, by Dosage

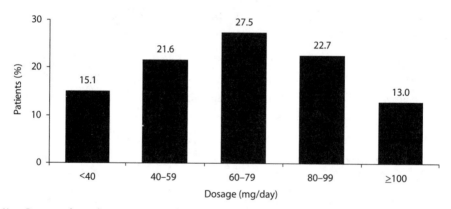

Note: Because of rounding, percentages do not sum to exactly 100.

The proportion of patients receiving dosages of less than 40 mg a day was significantly different for programs according to size; smaller MMT programs reported a higher percentage of patients at this dosage. This was also the case for dosages between 40 and 59 mg a day (Figure 6.2).

**Figure 6.2   Patients in Treatment at Least 2 Weeks Receiving
Maintenance Doses, by Dosage and Program Size**

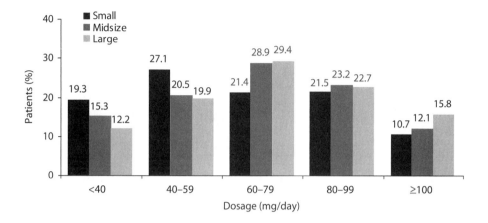

Note: Because of rounding, percentages do not sum to exactly 100. Small = 0–100 patients;
midsize = 101–300 patients; large = 301 or more patients.

The average maintenance dosage ranged from a minimum of 23 mg a day
to a maximum of 80 mg a day. Overall, the mean maintenance dosage across
all programs was 69 mg a day. As indicated by the findings presented in
Figure 6.3, small MMT programs reported a larger percentage of patients on
low maintenance dosages (less than 60 mg a day) compared with larger
programs, and there was no significant difference in dosing levels by either
organizational ownership or location.

Across programs, there was a broad range in the highest currently
prescribed maintenance dosage. The highest dosage offered in a for-profit
program was 1,100 mg a day, compared with 420 mg a day in a nonprofit/
public program. For-profit MMT programs had a larger average currently
prescribed maximum dosage (162 mg a day) than nonprofit/public programs
(140 mg a day; Figure 6.4). Large programs had a higher average maximum
dosage (182 mg a day) than midsize programs (137 mg a day) and small
programs (130 mg a day). The difference in mean highest currently prescribed
maintenance dosage was less pronounced among the large urban (152 mg a
day), urban (152 mg a day), and nonurban (133 mg a day) programs.

Figure 6.3   **Mean Maintenance Dosage for Patients in Treatment at Least 2 Weeks, by Program Ownership, Size, and Location**

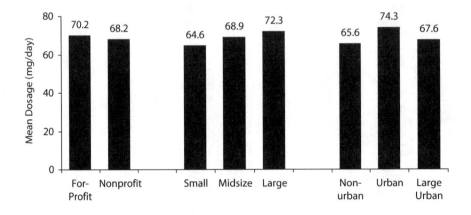

Figure 6.4   **Mean Maximum Dosage for Patients in Treatment at Least 2 Weeks, by Program Ownership, Size, and Location**

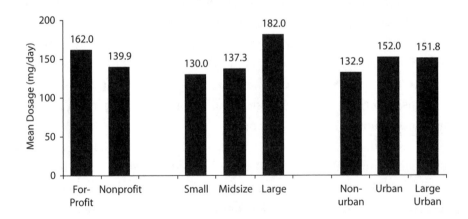

WHAT APPROACHES DO PHYSICIANS USE TO ESTABLISH DOSAGES?

Studies have documented that individuals currently in need of opiate dependence treatment are more varied by demographic characteristics than MMT patients in the past (Chatham et al., 1999; Craddock et al., 1981;

Wechsberg et al, 1998). Long-term comprehensive treatment, including medication and counseling, may be required for patients; however, dosages need to be individualized according to how patients present and respond to MMT, taking into account metabolic differences (Leavitt, Shinderman, Maxwell, Eap, & Paris, 2000).

The NIH Consensus Statement recommended that a dosage of 60 mg a day may be sufficient to meet this criterion but suggested that some patients may need higher dosages (NIH, 1997). In addition, individual differences in the absorption, metabolism, and elimination of methadone supports the notion that professional discretion based on observation and patient reactions should be a primary factor in the determination of dosage (Rettig & Yarmolinsky, 1995).

The dosage of methadone an individual receives should be based on the clinical judgment of a physician trained to administer methadone (Ball & Ross, 1991; CSAT, 1999; DHHS, 2001a; National Institutes of Health [NIH], 1997; Parrino, 1993; Rettig & Yarmolinsky, 1995). Physicians in MMT programs typically determine patient dosages by conducting an initial medical examination. The content and comprehensiveness of this initial examination can vary by program, as can individual treatment program policies with regard to determining maximum dosages.

The majority of physicians in the Evaluation Study (89%) reported that they determined dosages with patient feedback. Additionally, 86% of physicians reported that medical discretion (i.e., decisions based on physician input) was the main factor in determining the maximum dosage of methadone prescribed in a program.

WHAT ARE TAKE-HOME PRIVILEGES?

Take-home privileges allow patients in MMT to leave programs with one or more days' worth of their prescribed daily doses of methadone. For example, many MMT programs do not have operating clinical hours on Sundays. Therefore, on admission to treatment, each patient is allowed one take-home dose a week—the dose for Sunday. Other MMT programs operate 7 days a week and allow take-home doses only for patients who meet certain clinical criteria.

The FDA regulations stipulate that physicians must take into account the following criteria before granting take-home privileges: (1) absence of recent abuse of drugs (opiates, nonopiates, and alcohol), (2) regular clinic attendance, (3) absence of serious behavioral problems at the site, (4) absence of known criminal activity, (5) stability of the home environment and social relationships, (6) assurance that take-home medication can be safely stored, (7) assurance that the rehabilitative benefit to the patient outweighs the risk of diversion, and (8) length of time in MMT. Before granting take-home privileges, physicians are required to document these criteria in patients' medical charts.

The FDA regulations regarding the schedule and supply of take-home medications are as follows:

- After daily observation for the initial 3 months of treatment, patients can receive 2 days of take-home medication per week for the next 2 years in treatment.

- If patients continue to comply with program regulations for 3 years, they are allowed 3 days of take-home medication per week.

- After 3 years, patients can be granted weekly take-home privileges of 6 days of medication.

- Take-home privileges are not permitted for patients with a daily dose greater than 100 mg.

In reviewing these federal regulations, the committee members serving IOM supported much of the current policy; however, the committee regarded FDA's scheduling and supply regulations as too restrictive (Rettig & Yarmolinsky, 1995). Accordingly, IOM made the following recommendations:

- In the first month of treatment, patients visit the program six times a week and are limited to 1 day of take-home medication per week.

- In the second month, patients visit the program a minimum of three times a week and receive a maximum of 2 days of take-home medication per week.

- In the third month, patients come to the program at least twice a week and are given a maximum of 3 days of take-home medication per week.

- During the rest of the first year, patients visit the program at least once weekly and are given a maximum of 6 days of take-home medication per week.

- Thereafter, patients can visit the program monthly and can be given a maximum of 31 days of take-home medication.

In reviewing these recommendations, CSAT (1999) concurred with IOM on the behavioral criteria and documentation of decision making by the physician. However, CSAT changed the time criteria to the following schedule (CSAT, 2001):

- During the initial 90-day treatment period, patients are allowed a maximum of one unsupervised dose per week.

- During the second 90-day treatment period, patients are allowed a maximum of two unsupervised doses per week.

- During the third 90-day treatment period, patients are allowed a maximum of three unsupervised doses per week.

- During the remainder of treatment years 1 and 2, patients are allowed a maximum of six unsupervised doses per week.

- For year 3 of treatment and beyond, patients are allowed a maximum of 30 unsupervised doses per month.

The Final Rule supplemented CSAT's time criteria with the following provision (DHHS, 2001a): after 1 year of continuous treatment, patients may be given a maximum 2-week supply of take-home medication.

WHO MAKES THE DECISION FOR A PATIENT TO RECEIVE TAKE-HOME PRIVILEGES?

As discussed in the previous answer, the Final Rule includes increased schedule flexibility for medications dispensed to patients for unsupervised use, including provisions that permit up to a 30-day supply (DHHS, 2001). According to the Final Rule and CSAT's accreditation guidelines (2001), take-home privileges are determined by a multidisciplinary team, typically led by the primary clinician with direct oversight by a medical director. Physicians are called on to exercise professional discretion in determining eligibility (in accordance with established criteria and time frames). Furthermore, physicians must monitor patients receiving medications for unsupervised use by reviewing physician take-home decisions at least every 90 days and documenting these reviews in patient charts. Such reviews must evaluate drug testing results and other relevant clinical factors. The CSAT guidelines state that "physicians must be aware of the physiological issues, differences among laboratories, and factors that impact absorption, metabolism, and elimination of opiates" (2001, p. 20). Thus, as the time frame and supply guidelines for take-home privileges become less stringent, it is incumbent on physicians to be well educated about the physiological and behavioral aspects of opiate dependence treatment before exercising their professional discretion.

HOW MANY PATIENTS RECEIVE TAKE-HOME PRIVILEGES?

The Evaluation Study examined take-home medication practices by using two survey items that required program directors to list the number of patients in treatment less than and more than a year with no privileges and with 1-day, 2-day, or 3-day or more take-home privileges each week.

As shown in Figure 6.5, the majority of patients in MMT for less than a year did not receive take-home privileges. Of those who did, the proportion of patients with three or more take-home doses a week was higher than the proportions of those with one or two take-home doses a week. This finding remained true for patients in treatment for more than a year.

The proportion of patients in treatment longer than a year who had no take-home privileges was about 30% lower (i.e., 40% for patients in treatment more than a year versus 69% for patients in treatment less than a year) than for patients in treatment less than a year. Proportions for take-home privileges of one and two times a week were slightly higher for the patients in treatment longer than a year. The proportion of patients in treatment longer than a year who had take-home privileges of three or more times a week was substantially greater than for those in treatment less than a year.

There were no significant differences in proportions of take-home privileges for patients in treatment longer than a year, according to program ownership status, size, or location.

As shown in Table 6.1, with regard to patients in treatment less than a year, for-profit programs had almost twice as many patients with three or more take-home medications per week (20%) as the nonprofit/public programs (11%).

Figure 6.5 Patients Receiving Take-Home Privileges, by Time in Treatment (%)

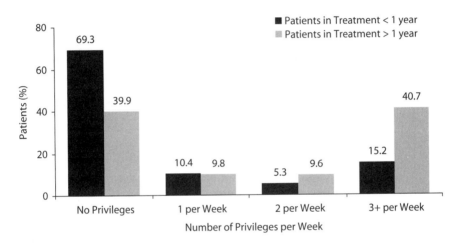

WHAT IS DIVERSION?

Methadone diversion is when methadone is not taken by the intended patient but rather is sold or shared. DEA has established MMT regulations and procedures to help prevent diversion. In addition to registering all practitioners who dispense methadone, DEA reviews programs for compliance with regulations about physical security, storage of narcotics, dispensing of narcotics, and maintenance of records and inventories of narcotic substances. Because of these responsibilities, DEA's role in regulating MMT did not change with the implementation of new federal clinical guidelines and regulations.

Table 6.1   Patients Receiving Take-Home Privileges, by Time in
             Treatment and Program Ownership, Size, and Location

	Program (%)							
	Ownership		Size			Location		
	For-Profit	Non-profit	Small	Mid-size	Large	Non-urban	Urban	Large Urban
In Treatment < 1 year								
No privileges	65.1	73.0	67.3	69.6	70.2	63.9	67.8	70.6
1 per week	10.4	10.4	10.7	8.5	13.2	13.6	8.6	10.7
2 per week	4.5	6.0	4.7	5.6	5.2	3.0	7.3	4.8
3+ per week	20.2	10.7	17.7	16.3	11.4	19.5	16.3	14.1
In Treatment > 1 year								
No privileges	37.3	41.1	37.8	37.4	45.3	40.7	33.4	42.2
1 per week	10.0	9.7	8.0	10.0	10.6	7.2	9.3	10.3
2 per week	8.3	10.7	9.7	10.2	8.6	11.4	11.2	8.8
3+ per week	44.5	37.5	44.5	42.4	35.5	40.7	46.1	38.7

Note: Because of rounding, percentages do not sum to exactly 100. Small = 0–100 patients;
midsize = 101–300 patients; large = 301 or more patients.

According to a 1995 DEA report about methadone diversion, which was
written in response to the IOM report, the nature of diversion has been
consistent and constant (Rettig & Yarmolinsky, 1995). Diversion generally
occurs under circumstances where the law is difficult to enforce (e.g., take-
home doses) and through lax program procedures. By citing cases of theft
and robbery over the past two decades, DEA demonstrated concern that the
risks associated with methadone diversion would increase under less restrictive regulations.

The Final Rule recognizes DEA's concerns and states that diversion
prevention is a critical aspect of the FDA regulatory system and must be
adequately addressed in any new system (DHHS, 2001a). The rule emphasizes, however, the changing environment of opiate treatment over time.

Under the CSAT regulatory guidelines and standards, MMT programs are required to develop a diversion control plan as a mechanism of their overall quality assurance.

This new requirement shifts responsibility for preventing diversion from the external inspections required under the FDA system directly to treatment programs. MMT programs are required to implement diversion control in their operating practices as outlined in an internal quality assurance and control plan.

All the MMT programs surveyed had preventive measures in place to discourage diversion. The most widely used deterrent (100% of the programs) was observing patients as they took their methadone dose. As another deterrent, 96% of the programs routinely made their patients aware of the risks and consequences of diverting methadone. About 86% relied on management staff to review or monitor dispensing records. Many programs (86%) used systematic observation of site environs to discourage diversion, and 96% prohibited loitering on site premises. Several programs listed other methods to discourage the methadone diversion, including the following:

- locked boxes for take-home dosing
- rare takeouts
- recalls of take-home doses
- reliance on word of mouth
- take-home bottle return policy
- committee review of incidents of diversion
- urine testing for methadone

Patient responses and urinalysis logs showed the extent of diversion to be minimal. The mean percentage of patients in a given MMT program reporting having seen other patients from their program selling or trading methadone doses in the past 3 months was 12%, with a range of 0 to 50% of patients at a program reporting having observed diversion. This measure is difficult to interpret, however, because it is not known whether higher proportions of patients observing diversion mean that there was more diversion at a program, or whether more patients observed a single act of diversion. That is, the extent to which diversion is observed may be a poor indicator of the actual extent of diversion in a program.

The mean proportion of patients who tested negative for methadone in their urine was about 2%, with a range of 0 to 50%. This measure should also be interpreted with caution. Although the on-site data collection team made every effort to exclude new patients from urinalysis data abstraction, it may be that some cases of methadone-negative urinalysis results were from new patients who had not yet begun treatment. Additionally, individuals synthesize methadone at different rates; a proportion of negative urine results may therefore be false negatives, requiring caution in how they are interpreted.

HOW DO MMT DIRECT CARE STAFF PREVENT METHADONE DIVERSION?

DEA has its own set of regulations and procedures with regard to opiate treatment programs, especially for diversion and security of narcotics. In addition to registering all practitioners who use methadone, DEA reviews treatment programs for compliance with regulations about physical security, storage of narcotics, dispensing of narcotics, and maintenance of records and inventories of narcotic substances. The Evaluation Study focused on MMT program administrative policies and procedures addressing punitive action for suspected diversion, administrative policies discouraging diversion activities, and take-home policies.

Two binary variables were computed to condense the program policy variables into single indicators. One variable, called "strict policies," was scored yes if

- a program reported that it typically relied on more than one method to discourage diversion,

- discharge was likely or extremely likely for diversion or attempted diversion, and

- the program frequently or always revoked take-home dosing for suspected diversion.

The other variable, called "strictest policies," was scored yes if

- a program reported that it typically relied on more than one method to discourage diversion,
- discharge was extremely likely for diversion or attempted diversion, and
- the program always revoked take-home dosing privileges for suspected diversion.

About 36% of the programs were categorized as having strict policies, and only 16% were categorized as having strictest policies.

More specifically, most of the MMT programs (about 87%) indicated that they relied on strict policies recommending or requiring patient discharge for methadone diversion. Almost 50% of the programs indicated that early discharge (i.e., discharge before completing treatment) was extremely likely for attempted diversion; an additional 34% indicated that discharge was likely. The likelihood of early discharge for successful diversion was somewhat greater: 77% indicated that it was extremely likely, and 14% indicated that it was likely. When asked how frequently the staff revoked take-home privileges if a patient was suspected of diverting methadone, 40% of the programs indicated that privileges were always revoked, 26% indicated that privileges were frequently revoked, and about 7% indicated that privileges were never revoked.

Table 6.2 presents the distribution of two key variables capturing the extent of diversion and two summary measures capturing the strictness of policies, by program size, ownership, and urbanicity. No statistically significant differences were found with either of the summary measures (for strict policies or strictest policies), suggesting that efforts to discourage diversion did not vary significantly across program types. Looking at the extent of observed diversion, we see that patients at larger programs were more likely to report having observed diversion. Almost 17% of patients from the largest programs reported having seen someone selling or trading their methadone dose, compared with about 12% at the midsize programs and about 6% at the smallest programs. Again, this finding should be interpreted with caution, as the difference may not be in the number of diversion episodes seen by patients, but rather in the number of patients reporting seeing the same episode.

Table 6.2 Methadone Diversion in MMT Programs

	Patients (mean %)		Programs (%)	
	Who Observed Diversion	With Urinalysis Results Negative for Methadone	With Strict Policies	With Strictest Policies
Overall	12.1	2.4	35.5	15.8
Ownership				
For-profit	9.9	2.2	28.6	11.9
Nonprofit/public	14.1	2.7	41.5	19.1
Size				
Small	5.8	3.5	28.4	11.3
Midsize	11.7	2.4	38.7	23.1
Large	16.9	1.9	35.4	7.7
Urbanicity				
Nonurban	7.7	4.1	29.0	14.5
Urban	11.8	1.9	31.7	24.0
Large urban	12.8	2.4	37.8	12.9

Note: Small = 1–100 patients; midsize = 101–300 patients; large = 301 or more patients.

WHAT IS METHADONE-ASSOCIATED MORTALITY?

The term *methadone-associated mortality* refers to recorded deaths in which methadone has been detected by a coroner or medical examiner. The task of defining the role of methadone in fatalities is complicated by inconsistencies in methods of determining and reporting causes of death, the presence of other central nervous system drugs, and the absence of information about individuals' substance use history and tolerance.

Concerns about the safety of methadone have been exacerbated in recent years as deaths related to methadone overdose have become more common in some areas. In certain regions of the country, methadone overdose has a higher incidence than, for example, overdose from OxyContin and other opioid pain medications. The increase in methadone overdoses has drawn the most attention in relation to the deaths of young drug users for whom methadone has not been prescribed. In most of these cases, the attributed cause has not been the diversion of liquid methadone from MMT programs (e.g., through theft or sale of take-home doses); rather, it has been the diversion of wafer or pill forms of methadone prescribed as a long-term treatment for severe, chronic pain.

Because methadone does not produce euphoria, users who are familiar with other opiates (which produce a more intense high with each additional dose) may decide to take larger doses in pursuit of intoxication. Larger doses of methadone administered to a methadone-naïve individual can be lethal. This problem is also faced by physicians in MMT clinics who must strike a delicate balance between use of the maximum initial dosage to ensure treatment retention and use of the minimum initial dosage to avoid complications or fatality. Most of the MMT patients who experience methadone overdose do so during the induction period, occasionally when physicians have failed to strike this balance but also when patients are using drugs in addition to methadone (Srivastava & Kahan, 2006). Avoiding fatalities caused by diversion of methadone, as by induction overdose and drug interaction, involves the establishment of close relationships between MMT physicians and patients. Such relationships facilitate communication between doctors and patients and enable close monitoring of patients' progress. Where patient-to-staff ratios are high, however, it can be difficult to establish this kind of relationship.

Although an in-depth examination of methadone-associated mortality is beyond the scope of this book, SAMHSA convened a multidisciplinary group to conduct the National Assessment of Methadone-Associated Mortality in May 2003. The findings and recommendations from SAMHSA's national assessment were published in 2004 and are available through SAMHSA's National Clearinghouse (http://www.health.org/).

SUMMARY

- The average maintenance dosage ranged from 23 to 80 mg a day, with a mean of 69 mg.

- Differences were found by program size and ownership in dosage patterns. For-profit and larger programs had a higher mean maximum dosage.

- Smaller and less urban programs had slightly lower mean dosages.

- The majority of patients in treatment less than a year had no take-home privileges.

- Almost 41% of patients had three or more take-home privileges after being in treatment longer than a year.

CHAPTER 7—The Costs and Funding of Methadone Maintenance Treatment

With limited resources to allocate to competing health interventions, policy makers and payers are increasingly concerned about accountability for resources expended in providing substance abuse treatment (Zarkin, Dunlap, Bray, & Wechsberg, 2002). Measures such as total costs, cost per patient, and service unit costs are important indicators of resource use. An evaluation of treatment costs can provide valuable insight about the inputs needed for treatment provision and help guide policy makers and providers in allocating resources efficiently.

Treatment funding is also important to the overall understanding of treatment provision. Funding of substance abuse treatment, especially MMT, differs from funding of other health care services because of the dominant role of public agencies as payers (Horgan & Merrick, 2001). In recent years, significant changes in funding mechanisms have occurred, including the growth of managed care practices among both private and public funding sources and the introduction of accreditation, which may affect eligibility for certain funding. Information on funding provides a more complete picture of MMT provision, including which funding resources may be available for treatment and how these scarce resources can be drawn together from various government agencies, private entities, and individual patients so that treatment can be provided effectively.

This chapter presents a review of total costs, per-patient costs, and costs for specific services, as well as a descriptive analysis of funding for MMT programs. The Evaluation Study provided a unique opportunity to examine both costs and funding for MMT programs nationwide. Cost and funding data from 170 MMT programs were collected over 2 years.[1] Each treatment

---

[1] Two programs that participated in the larger Evaluation Study were excluded from the economic evaluation because they were not independent outpatient sites, as initially reported, but were embedded within a larger therapeutic community and residential facility. It was decided that their organizational structure and costs were too different from those of the other outpatient MMT settings and that their inclusion would bias the average cost estimates.

program was asked to provide cost and funding data for its most recently completed fiscal year. Differences in fiscal years reported across programs resulted in economic data for different fiscal years: 1997 (5% of the evaluation sample), 1998 (61%), and 1999 (34%). All cost and funding dollars were adjusted to year 2000 dollars. The cost methodology and results were presented in Zarkin, Dunlap, and Homsi (2004).

HOW MUCH DOES MMT COST?

The estimated total annual cost for MMT programs in year 2000 dollars was $924,748. The estimated annual cost per patient was $4,176, a finding comparable to other cost estimates reported in the literature, which range from approximately $2,800 to $6,300 (figures in year 2000 dollars; Zarkin et al., 2004). The cost estimation took an economic perspective; therefore, these estimates include the value of donated or subsidized resources, such as volunteer labor and subsidized building space, as well as actual expenditures paid by the programs. According to this perspective, the treatment program and cost estimates do not include the value of resources used by other involved parties, such as patients and government agencies. Zarkin et al. provided a detailed description of the cost estimation methodology.

To gain a better understanding of these costs, the average annual total cost and average annual cost per patient were examined by selected program characteristics—organizational ownership (i.e., for-profit versus nonprofit/public), program size, urbanicity of location, and organizational structure (i.e., whether programs had a parent organization)—to determine whether treatment costs differed by key program characteristics. Table 7.1 presents cost estimates for the total annual cost and annual cost per patient, by program characteristics.

As shown, average annual per-patient costs varied little across the subgroups. The estimated average per-patient cost of $4,580 for nonprofit/public programs was not significantly different from the for-profit cost of $3,713. Thus, per-patient annual costs among nonprofit/public and for-profit programs were very similar. Smaller treatment programs tended to have greater annual costs per patient, compared with larger programs. The average per-patient cost was $5,216 for programs with 1 to 100 patients, compared with $3,812 for programs with over 300 patients. These findings suggest that larger programs may benefit from some economies of scale in providing treatment. The estimated average cost per patient was not significantly different for programs in areas with a population less than 250,000, compared with programs in more densely populated areas. However, programs belonging to a parent organization had significantly greater costs than independent programs ($4,575 versus $3,229).

Table 7.1 Average Annual Costs (2000$), by MMT Program Characteristics

	Costs ($)	
	Total	**Per Patient per Year**
Overall	$924,748	$4,176
Ownership		
For-profit	$766,989	$3,713
Nonprofit/public	$1,062,467	$4,580
Size		
Small	$286,402	$5,216
Midsize	$681,193	$3,996
Large	$1,671,823	$3,812
Urbanicity		
Nonurban	$311,633	$3,504
Urban	$735,212	$4,056
Large urban	$1,061,103	$4,293
Parent Organization		
Yes	$1,010,461	$4,575
No	$721,278	$3,229

Note: Small = 1–100 patients; midsize = 101–300 patients; large = 301 or more patients. Data were weighted in all analyses.

Source: Zarkin et al., 2004; Wechsberg et al., 2003.

WHAT ARE THE COSTS OF SPECIFIC MMT SERVICES?

Although total cost and cost per patient are important measures of overall resource use in providing treatment, they are limited because they do not provide information on the costs for specific treatment services. This information is becoming increasingly important for providers as focus shifts from aggregated total costs to more specific service-level evaluations. As funding from entities that use service reimbursement structures (e.g., private health insurance) increases, MMT providers need cost information at the service level to help guide them in their resource allocation. In addition, as noted by an IOM report (Rettig & Yarmolinsky, 1995), programs should offer services that are needed most by patients, but funding scarcity requires that these services also be cost-effective. Therefore, programs need information on costs and resource use at the service level rather than simply at the aggregate annual level.

To estimate the average unit cost for specific MMT services, the Evaluation Study used information on the total costs incurred by a program and the program's labor allocation across various treatment services and program activities. Zarkin et al. (2004) provided a detailed description of the methods used in the service-level cost estimation.

The service-level cost estimates include the costs for labor and nonlabor resources used in the direct provision of specific treatment services and the labor and nonlabor costs of related administrative activities and other indirect services. Nonlabor resources include building space, contracted services, supplies and materials, miscellaneous resources (e.g., utilities, communication costs), and overhead or administrative costs incurred for services provided at the level of a parent organization (e.g., human resources, legal services, billing). Labor resources include the time spent by clinics in the direct provision of treatment and the time spent by staff in related activities necessary for providing treatment and maintaining clinic operations, such as administrative activities, QA, and program evaluation performed within the program.

Table 7.2 presents average cost estimates for specific MMT services. A session of initial patient assessment and treatment planning was the most costly, with average costs of approximately $106 per session. Direct labor accounted for 41% of these costs. Time spent per session of initial planning assessment and treatment planning varied by program, with an average of 111 minutes per session. This time variation translates into large variation across programs in the costs of providing this service.

Less variation was found among programs for the costs of individual and group counseling sessions. Individual counseling sessions lasted 43 minutes on average. The average cost for an individual counseling session was approximately $36 per patient. On average, group counseling sessions lasted 77 minutes. The average cost of a group counseling session was approximately $9 per patient, and the cost per session depended on the number of patients (the average number of patients per group counseling session was nine). Direct labor accounted for approximately 36% of the total costs of individual counseling and 37% of the total costs of group counseling.

Table 7.2   Average Service-Level Costs per Patient (2000$)

Service	Service Unit	Per Patient Per Service Unit		
		Average Time (min)	Direct Labor Cost	Total Cost
Initial patient assessment and treatment planning	Session	110.6	$43.41	$105.95
Initial medical services	Session	61.4	$46.90	$79.88
Individual counseling	Session	43.2	$12.79	$35.65
Group counseling	Session	76.7	$3.22	$8.59
Methadone dosing	Week	21.8	$7.44	$24.29
Ongoing medical services	Week	6.9	$3.77	$7.53
Case management	Week	11.7	$3.58	$10.22
QA	Week	8.5	$3.32	$7.94

Source: Zarkin et al., 2004.

Several treatment services did not have clearly defined sessions. For example, case management includes many different kinds of activities that help facilitate treatment recovery. A session might include a 15-minute phone call regarding a referral to another social service agency or a 2-hour meeting with a patient to discuss housing options. Because defining mean-ingful sessions for these treatment services is not possible, the cost per patient per week was estimated. The costs of these services ranged from $8 (ongoing medical services) to $24 (methadone dosing) per patient per week. Direct labor accounted for 35% to 50% of total costs.

As with total and per-patient costs, the study examined differences in service-level costs by selected program characteristics. The estimated costs of providing a session of initial patient assessment differed by ownership and organizational structure (Table 7.3). The average total cost per session was greater for nonprofit/public programs than for for-profit programs. This result is explained in part by the greater average time spent per patient in nonprofit/public programs. In addition, programs that were part of a parent organization had a significantly greater average cost for an initial patient assessment, compared with programs that were not.

Table 7.3 Average Time and Costs per Session for Initial Patient Assessment, by MMT Program Characteristics (2000$), n=160

	Per Session		
	Average Time (min)	Direct Labor Cost	Total Cost
Ownership			
For-profit, n=69	93.5	$33.79	$82.86
Nonprofit/public, n=91	126.9	$52.54	$127.88
Size			
Small, n=32	99.6	$35.49	$87.53
Midsize, n=79	110.9	$41.89	$101.54
Large, n=49	117.1	$50.66	$124.17
Urbanicity			
Nonurban, n=13	109.8	$43.36	$95.86
Urban, n=40	117.6	$41.96	$101.26
Large urban, n=107	108.1	$43.95	$108.89
Parent Organization			
Yes, n=111	117.8	$48.69	$118.99
No, n=49	94.6	$31.50	$76.59

Note: Small = 1–100 patients; midsize = 101–300 patients; large = 301 or more patients.

Similar cost differences were found for initial medical services. As shown in Table 7.4, nonprofit/public programs had a greater average cost for an initial medical service session, compared with for-profit programs ($89 versus $70). Again, some of this difference is explained by the greater average time spent per patient by nonprofit/public programs in providing initial medical services. Programs that were part of a parent organization also had significant greater costs for an initial medical service session, compared with programs that were not ($85 versus $69). Costs for initial medical service sessions did not differ significantly by program size or urbanicity.

Table 7.4   Average Time and Costs per Session for Initial Medical Services, by Program Characteristics (2000$), n=157

	Per Session		
	Average Time (min)	Direct Labor Cost	Total Cost
Ownership			
For-profit, n=67	53.9	$42.68	$69.96
Nonprofit/public, n=90	68.5	$50.87	$89.14
Size			
Small, n=32	62.9	$48.98	$80.72
Midsize, n=78	59.9	$45.81	$76.05
Large, n=47	62.8	$47.31	$85.35
Urbanicity			
Nonurban, n=13	71.3	$53.77	$91.53
Urban, n=38	64.9	$43.67	$72.99
Large urban, n=106	59.0	$47.28	$80.98
Parent Organization			
Yes, n=109	63.6	$49.01	$84.74
No, n=48	56.6	$42.24	$69.01

Note: Small = 1–100 patients; midsize = 101–300 patients; large = 301 or more patients.

The costs for an individual counseling session (Table 7.5) did not differ by ownership or organizational structure. However, there were significant differences by program size and urbanicity.

The only significant cost difference found for group counseling sessions was between programs in nonurban areas and those in large urban areas. Programs in nonurban areas had greater per-patient group counseling costs, compared with programs in large urban areas ($10.97 versus $8.99).

Table 7.5   Average Time and Costs per Session for Individual Counseling, by Program Characteristics (2000$), n=165

	Per Session		
	Average Time (min)	Direct Labor Cost	Total Cost
Ownership			
For-profit, n=68	44.3	$12.05	$33.89
Nonprofit/public, n=97	42.2	$13.45	$37.20
Size			
Small, n=32	46.9	$14.09	$39.73
Midsize, n=82	45.9	$13.12	$36.60
Large, n=51	36.7	$11.53	$31.78
Urbanicity			
Nonurban, n=13	43.0	$13.12	$37.05
Urban, n=42	40.3	$11.40	$29.99
Large urban, n=110	54.8	$14.59	$42.36
Parent Organization			
Yes, n=116	43.3	$13.16	$37.07
No, n=49	42.9	$11.92	$32.32

Note: Small = 1–100 patients; midsize = 101–300 patients; large = 301 or more patients.

As shown in Table 7.6, weekly per-patient costs for ongoing medical services were greater for programs that were part of a parent organization than for programs that were not ($8 versus $6 per patient per week), and weekly per-patient costs for ongoing medical services were less for programs that were located in nonurban areas, compared with programs in either urban or large urban areas. The study found no significant differences in ongoing medical services by program ownership or size.

Table 7.6   Average Time and Costs per Patient per Week for Ongoing Medical Services, by MMT Program Characteristics (2000$), n=164

	Per Session		
	Average Time (min)	Direct Labor Cost	Total Cost
Ownership			
For-profit, n=67	6.3	$3.37	$6.43
Nonprofit/public, n=97	7.3	$4.11	$8.48
Size			
Small, n=31	9.1	$4.43	$9.31
Midsize, n=82	6.5	$3.47	$6.81
Large, n=51	6.1	$3.84	$7.62
Urbanicity			
Nonurban, n=12	4.3	$2.07	$4.04
Urban, n=42	7.0	$3.24	$6.70
Large urban, n=110	7.0	$4.15	$8.21
Parent Organization			
Yes, n=115	7.2	$4.14	$8.32
No, n=49	6.1	$2.92	$5.70

Note: Small = 1–100 patients; midsize = 101–300 patients; large = 301 or more patients.

There were similar differences for the weekly per-patient costs of case management. As shown in Table 7.7, programs that were part of a parent organization had significant greater per-patient case management costs, compared with programs that were not ($12 versus $6 per patient per week). Programs in nonurban areas had lower weekly per-patient case management costs, compared with programs in large urban areas ($6 versus $10 per patient per week).

Table 7.7   Average Time and Costs per Patient per Week for Case Management Services, by MMT Program Characteristics (2000$), n=147

	Per Patient Per Week		
	Average Time (min)	Direct Labor Cost	Total Cost
Ownership			
For-profit, n=60	13.4	$3.57	$11.08
Nonprofit/public, n=87	10.2	$3.58	$9.49
Size			
Small, n=26	14.0	$4.50	$11.06
Midsize, n=73	11.0	$3.14	$9.89
Large, n=48	11.5	$3.73	$10.27
Urbanicity			
Nonurban, n=11	8.6	$2.58	$6.34
Urban, n=38	14.8	$3.60	$12.82
Large urban, n=98	10.7	$3.67	$9.62
Parent Organization			
Yes, n=103	12.6	$4.02	$11.88
No, n=44	9.6	$2.56	$6.42

Note: Small = 1–100 patients; midsize = 101–300 patients; large = 301 or more patients.

No significant cost differences for methadone dosing were found by program ownership or urbanicity (Table 7.8). However, small programs had significant greater weekly per-patient methadone dosing costs than larger programs. Some of this difference is explained by the greater average time spent per patient per week in these programs. Programs that were part of a parent organization had greater weekly per-patient methadone dosing costs, compared with programs that were not ($26 versus $19 per patient per week).

Table 7.8 Average Time and Costs per Patient per Week for Methadone Dosing, by MMT Program Characteristics (2000$), n=165

	Per Patient Per Week		
	Average Time (min)	**Direct Labor Cost**	**Total Cost**
Ownership			
For-profit, n=69	20.5	$6.11	$21.71
Nonprofit/public, n=96	23.1	$8.64	$26.61
Size			
Small, n=33	33.7	$9.92	$33.04
Midsize, n=82	20.2	$7.05	$22.65
Large, n=50	17.0	$6.50	$21.33
Urbanicity			
Nonurban, n=13	28.0	$8.57	$28.42
Urban, n=42	21.7	$6.63	$22.55
Large urban, n=110	21.2	$7.62	$24.48
Parent Organization			
Yes, n=116	22.7	$8.07	$26.39
No, n=49	19.8	$5.97	$19.34

Note: Small = 1–100 patients; midsize = 101–300 patients; large = 301 or more patients.

Finally, there were significant differences in the average costs of QA between for-profit and nonprofit/public programs (Table 7.9), with greater average weekly per-patient costs at the nonprofit/public programs. There were also differences in average QA costs by urbanicity; programs in urban and large urban areas had greater average weekly per-patient costs for QA than programs in nonurban areas. Further, programs that were part of a parent organization had greater average weekly per-patient costs than programs that were not.

Table 7.9 Average Time and Costs per Patient per Week for QA, by MMT Program Characteristics (2000$)

	Per Patient Per Week		
	Average Time (min)	Direct Labor Cost	Total Cost
Ownership			
For-profit, n=67	7.2	$2.68	$6.36
Nonprofit/public, n=96	9.6	$3.87	$9.33
Size			
Small, n=32	12.4	$4.27	$10.00
Midsize, n=80	7.6	$2.99	$7.24
Large, n=51	7.4	$3.24	$7.78
Urbanicity			
Nonurban, n=12	6.0	$2.01	$5.12
Urban, n=41	8.8	$3.17	$7.77
Large urban, n=110	8.6	$3.51	$8.30
Parent Organization			
Yes, n=115	8.7	$3.51	$8.69
No, n=48	8.0	$2.86	$6.19

Note: Small = 1–100 patients; midsize = 101–300 patients; large = 301 or more patients.

HOW IS MMT FUNDED?

As part of the Evaluation Study, programs self-reported funding sources for their most recently completed fiscal year, and these sources were examined across four broad funding categories: public insurance, other public sources, patient fees, and other private sources. Public insurance included Medicaid, Medicare, and Civilian Health and Medical Program of the Uniformed Services (CHAMPUS) funding. Other public sources included all other government sources of funding, such as Substance Abuse Prevention and Treatment (SAPT) block grants, single state agencies, and state and local governments. Patient fees are those paid directly by patients out-of-pocket. Other private sources included funding from private insurance (e.g., managed care), foundations, or corporations.

The estimated annual MMT funding per patient per year was $4,018. Total funding for each program was calculated by summing the site-reported total funding for each funding category. The funding per patient per year represents a program's estimated total annual funding divided by the number of patients enrolled at the program on a given day (i.e., the average daily census). The majority of funding came from other public sources (e.g., SAPT block grants, single state agencies, state and local government; $1,525) and patient fees ($1,306). Other sources of program funding included public insurance ($1,060) and other private funds ($127).

The average annual total funding and average annual funding per patient were estimated by the same program characteristics as were costs—organizational ownership, program size, urbanicity, and organizational structure. As shown in Table 7.10, average per-patient funding varied little across the selected program characteristics. The only significant differences in per-patient annual funding were by ownership, size, and whether a program was part of a parent organization. On average, nonprofit/public programs reported greater per-patient funding than for-profit programs ($4,435 versus $3,539). For-profit programs received a greater amount of per-patient funding from patient fees than nonprofit/public programs. Conversely, nonprofit/public programs received a greater amount of per-patient funding from other public sources, compared with for-profit programs. Nonurban programs received a significantly smaller amount of funding from patient fees than more urban programs. Programs that were part of a parent organization reported greater per-patient funding than programs that were not ($4,296 versus $3,357).

Table 7.10　Average Annual Funding per Patient (2000$), by Program Characteristics

	Funding Category			
	Public Insurance	Other Public	Patient Fees	Other Private
Total	$1,060	$1,525	$1,306	$127
Ownership				
For-profit	$679	$579	$2,237	$44
Nonprofit/public	$1,392	$2,350	$493	$200
Size				
Small	$515	$1,865	$1,370	$289
Midsize	$937	$1,442	$1,563	$99
Large	$1,572	$1,440	$887	$71
Urbanicity				
Nonurban	$569	$1,897	$1,082	$28
Urban	$946	$1,118	$2,101	$114
Large urban	$1,155	$1,633	$1,039	$143
Parent Organization				
Yes	$1,229	$1,862	$1,070	$135
No	$658	$724	$1,866	$109

Note: Small = 1–100 patients; midsize = 101–300 patients; large = 301 or more patients.

SUMMARY

- The estimated annual cost per patient for MMT in year 2000 dollars was $4,176.

- Small programs have greater per-patient costs ($5,216) than midsize ($3,996) or large programs ($3,812).

- The estimated average cost for an initial patient assessment was $106 per session. The estimated average cost for an initial medical session was $80. For both of these services, the average session cost was greater in nonprofit/public programs because, in part, of the greater amount of time spent per patient per session.

- The cost of individual counseling did not differ by ownership or organizational structure, but small programs had a greater average time per session than did large programs.

- On average, for-profit programs received a greater portion of funding from patient fees than did nonprofit/public programs.

- Programs that were part of a parent organization reported greater per-patient funding.

CHAPTER 8—Direct Care Staff and Their Activities

The experience, education, and qualifications of treatment staff are integral to providing high-quality MMT. Although MMT has been available for decades, little is known about the staff of MMT programs. In this chapter, we present the characteristics, backgrounds, and perspectives of the direct care staff who work with patients in MMT.

WHO PROVIDES MMT SERVICES?

Providing high-quality treatment is interwoven with the experience, education, and qualifications of the treatment staff. Therefore, staff characteristics and activities have been a focus of best practices in MMT since its inception. MMT program staff typically include a clinical director and administrative personnel, counselors, case managers, intake workers, and medical personnel. The medical personnel may consist of a medical director or psychiatrist (responsible for administering all medical services), other physicians, physician assistants, and dosing nurses, depending on the size and needs of the MMT program.

Although MMT has been available for several decades, little is known about the demographic characteristics, experience, and workload of direct care staff at MMT programs. The Evaluation Study examined characteristics, backgrounds, and perspectives of direct care staff (i.e., staff working directly with patients), including counselors (persons with an active patient caseload) and physicians at the 172 MMT program sites included in the study.

The analyses focused on staff who worked directly with patients for all or part of their work week, including clinical supervisors, nurses, case managers, and intake workers. Further, because physicians have a special role within MMT programs and often are only part-time staff, they were surveyed using a separate instrument. Therefore, the Evaluation Study reported on them separately. An in-depth examination of how physicians spend their time was published in the *Journal of Addictive Diseases* (Wechsberg et al., 2004).

WHO ARE THE DIRECT CARE STAFF?

The study asked, "What are the characteristics of staff in a national sample of MMT programs?" Although MMT program staff can be categorized into three groups (administrative, counseling, and medical), many perform roles that cut across classifications. For example, some medical staff solely dispense methadone, whereas others spend a portion of their time providing other services directly to patients (e.g., counseling).

As shown in Figure 8.1, the majority (52%) of direct care staff identified themselves as counselors; nurses were the second largest group (26%). It was much less common across programs for staff to report being case managers, clinical supervisors, or intake workers.

Figure 8.1   Direct Care Staff at MMT Programs, by Position

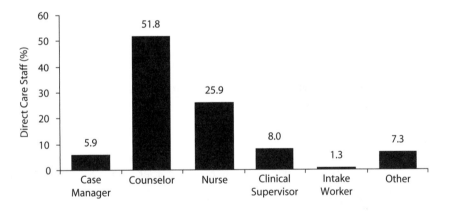

The majority of staff in all labor categories are female. Nurses, counselors, and clinical supervisors comprise the greatest percentage of female staff (Figure 8.2). The Evaluation Study found a higher percentage of female counselors than did Ball and Ross (1991; 58% versus 49%), perhaps reflecting changes over time in the makeup of the MMT workforce.

The Evaluation Study findings showed differences in direct care positions by the size and location of MMT programs (Table 8.1). At small MMT programs, a larger percentage of the staff were nurses and clinical supervisors, and a smaller percentage were counseling staff, compared with the staff of midsize and large MMT programs. These differences reflect the smaller patient census from these programs. Similar results were found in nonurban MMT programs.

Figure 8.2   Female Direct Care Staff at MMT Programs, by Position

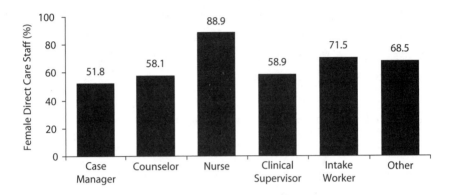

Table 8.1   Direct Care Positions at MMT Programs, by Program Size and Urbanicity

	Position (%)					
	Case Manager	**Counselor**	**Nurse**	**Clinical Supervisor**	**Intake Worker**	**Other**
Overall	5.9	51.8	25.9	8.0	1.3	7.3
Size						
Small	4.4	39.9	32.7	14.0	1.0	7.8
Midsize	5.6	48.9	27.4	8.1	1.2	8.8
Large	6.4	56.3	23.3	6.6	1.3	6.0
Urbanicity						
Nonurban	2.2	42.7	35.3	15.9	0.0	4.0
Urban	6.7	55.2	25.9	6.0	0.0	6.3
Large Urban	5.9	51.3	25.2	8.1	1.7	7.8

Note: Small = 1–100 patients; midsize = 101–300 patients; large = 301 or more patients.

ARE THERE STAFF DIFFERENCES BY RACE IN MMT?

Studies have shown that over half of MMT patients are White and male; however, the patient population also includes a sizeable proportion of African Americans and people of other races. Because many patients may relate better to staff from their own demographic group, it is important to examine the race of staff serving patients in MMT.

In all labor categories, the largest percentages of staff were either White or African American, and Whites were predominant across all labor categories (Figure 8.3). About 10% to 20% of direct care staff by position were Hispanic. These percentages differ slightly from the findings of Ball and Ross (1991), in which Whites and African Americans were represented equally across staff.

Figure 8.3   Race and Ethnicity of Direct Care Staff at MMT Programs, by Position

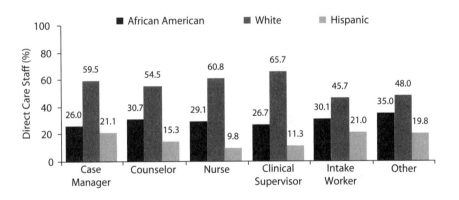

ARE THERE STAFF DIFFERENCES BY AGE?

The age distribution of staff differed significantly by position. The largest percentage of counselors, nurses, and clinical supervisors reported being between the ages of 45 and 54 (Table 8.2). The largest percentage of case managers and intake workers reported being between the ages of 25 and 34, reflecting that these positions were more likely to be considered entry level.

Table 8.2   Age of Direct Care Staff at MMT Programs, by Position, n=1,440

Position	Age (%)				
	18–24	25–34	35–44	45–54	55 or Older
Case manager	3.7	36.7	30.7	15.5	13.4
Counselor	4.9	26.3	24.7	32.8	11.4
Nurse	2.3	16.0	27.8	32.4	21.5
Clinical supervisor	1.1	12.8	34.6	40.0	11.6
Intake worker	11.6	41.2	22.2	25.0	0.0
Other	4.0	19.6	36.5	33.2	6.8

Note: Because of rounding error, rows may not sum to 100.

ARE THERE STAFF DIFFERENCES BY EDUCATIONAL LEVEL?

Recent studies by researchers in Australia have contributed to the growing interest in the impact of staff attitudes on the quality of care given to MMT patients (Calsyn et al., 1990; Caplehorn et al., 1998). Previous literature has observed that many MMT program policies are not consistent with best practices as proven through studies examining the effectiveness of MMT. This inconsistency between science and practice is often attributed to poor program administration and inadequate staff education or training. Because of these beliefs, the Evaluation Study researchers felt that it was imperative to examine staff differences in education and to further examine staff training.

The Evaluation Study found that education level varied significantly by direct care position (Table 8.3). Three-quarters of all nursing staff reported that their highest level of education was an associate's degree or less. These findings support the notion that nurses employed at MMT programs generally do not have advanced registered nurse (RN) degrees. In contrast, over half (56%) of the clinical supervisors reported having a master's degree or doctorate, and 64% of counselors had a bachelor's or master's degree. In contrast, Ball and Ross (1991) found that 34% of MMT program counselors reported having advanced degrees.

Table 8.3 Education Level of Direct Care Staff at MMT Programs, by Position, n=1,336

	Education Level (%)				
	HS Diploma/ GED	Associate's Degree	Bachelor's Degree	Master's Degree	Doctorate
Position					
Case manager	12.1	21.7	48.6	16.2	1.4
Counselor	19.0	15.8	35.7	28.5	1.1
Nurse	32.6	43.8	19.3	3.9	0.3
Clinical supervisor	10.2	10.4	23.4	48.9	7.0
Intake worker	22.4	6.0	41.8	29.9	0.0
Other	26.2	29.0	30.4	14.4	0.0

Note: GED=General Equivalency Diploma; HS=High school.

HOW MANY DIRECT CARE STAFF REPORT BEING IN RECOVERY?

There is some controversy about the value of employing recovering substance abusers at MMT programs. This controversy stems from growing professional and licensing requirements for a level of education that staff in recovery have often not achieved. Nonetheless, staff in recovery can play a vital role in the treatment process, not only as trained professionals but also as role models. In the Evaluation Study, about 17% of direct care staff were in recovery. This figure is only slightly higher than in the 1980s (11%) and slightly lower than Ball and Ross found (19%).

WHAT CERTIFICATIONS HAVE DIRECT CARE STAFF COMPLETED?

The Evaluation Study asked direct care staff about their current substance abuse certifications, including state certification, Certified Alcohol and Drug Abuse Counselor (CADAC), Certified Drug Abuse Counselor (CDAC), and Certified Addiction Counselor (CAC; Figure 8.4). Clinical supervisors represented the largest percentage of certified staff (64%), and case managers and counselors reported the next highest percentages (47% and 43%, respectively). Because only a small percentage of nurses maintain active patient caseloads, nurses were the least likely to have substance abuse certification; large and for-profit programs reported the smallest percentages of nurses with this type of certification. Certifications for this group, however, may not be as important as they are for other categories of direct care staff.

Figure 8.4   Substance Abuse Certifications Held by Direct Care MMT Staff

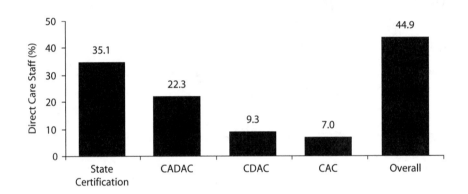

Note: CADAC=Certified Alcohol and Drug Abuse Counselor; CDAC=Certified Drug Abuse Counselor; CAC=Certified Addiction Counselor. Because multiple responses were allowed, percentages do not sum to 100.

Although certification and licensing have been a part of professionalizing the substance abuse field, only a small percentage of programs required staff to be certified, and less than half of the staff with a caseload had any form of substance abuse certification (Figure 8.4). This finding may suggest the need for incentives to encourage programs and their staff to pursue credentialing.

WHO ARE THE PHYSICIANS PROVIDING MMT SERVICES?

Studies examining the effectiveness of MMT have found positive associations between maximum methadone dose and retention in MMT programs. Despite this evidence, however, staff in many MMT programs continue to provide patients with inadequate doses of methadone and time-limited MMT (Caplehorn et al., 1998). It has been suggested that the underlying attitudes and belief systems of the individual physician can play a pivotal role in the successful outcomes of treatment for patients in MMT programs. It is therefore important to more fully understand who the physicians are who provide medical services in MMT programs.

Overall, 244 physicians practicing or working in MMT programs participated in the Evaluation Study. Physicians were primarily males; almost two-thirds (63%) were White, and about 7% were Hispanic (Figure 8.5). No physicians in the study were younger than 25, and three-quarters were aged 45 or older.

Figure 8.5 Physicians Practicing in MMT Programs, by Gender and Race

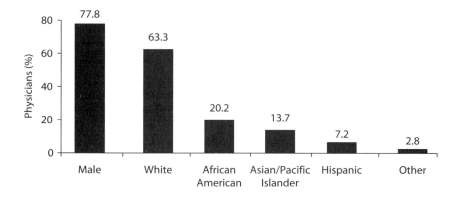

Only 17 (10%) of the 172 MMT programs in the Evaluation Study reported having a full-time physician/psychiatrist on staff. Large programs (12 of the 17 programs) in large urban locations (15 of the 17 programs) were the most likely to have a full-time physician/psychiatrist. Nonprofit or public organizations (11 of the 17 programs) were more likely than for-profit programs to have one.

HOW LONG HAVE DIRECT CARE STAFF AND PHYSICIANS WORKED IN SUBSTANCE ABUSE TREATMENT IN GENERAL AND MMT IN PARTICULAR?

Evaluation Study results showed that the number of years direct care staff and physicians had worked in substance abuse treatment varied greatly. Direct care staff, who included clinical supervisors, counselors, case managers, and intake workers, reported less experience in substance abuse treatment than the physicians employed by the MMT programs (Figure 8.6). Nearly half of the physicians (47%) reported more than 10 years of experience in substance abuse treatment, compared with only 25% of direct care staff. Among the direct care staff, clinical supervisors had the most substance abuse treatment experience; 22% reported more than 10 years. Nurses also had more substance abuse treatment experience; 39% had 6 years or more. In contrast, 56% of case managers and 63% of intake workers had 2 years or less of substance abuse treatment experience.

Figure 8.6   Years of Experience in Substance Abuse Treatment for Direct Care Staff and Physicians

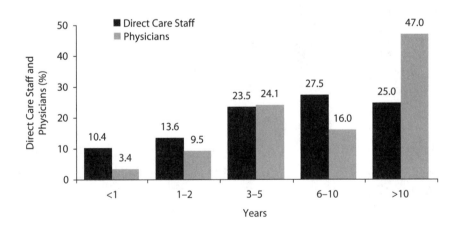

About a third (33%) of physicians reported working in MMT for more than 10 years, compared with only 12% of direct care staff (Figure 8.7). Only 6% of physicians had less than 1 year of experience in MMT, compared with

25% of direct care staff. Overall, although the vast majority of physicians were not employed full-time by the MMT programs, they reported having significantly more experience in both substance abuse treatment and MMT than all direct care staff.

Figure 8.7 Years of Experience in MMT for Direct Care Staff and Physicians

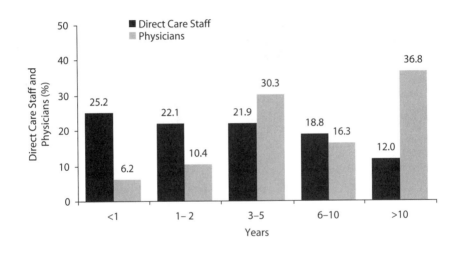

HOW DO MMT PROGRAM STAFF SPEND THEIR TIME?

Determining how MMT program staff spend their time can be important in assessing the quality of care provided (D'Aunno & Vaughn, 1995; Magura et al., 1999). The Evaluation Study surveyed direct care staff about the percentage of their counseling sessions that were with individuals versus groups and about the typical length of sessions. Across labor categories, most counseling sessions were with individual patients, and individual sessions lasted an average of 30 to 40 minutes. The length of group sessions varied by position, most likely reflecting the different emphases of groups led by different types of staff. For example, groups with counselors lasted, on average, about 45 minutes, whereas groups with nurses lasted closer to 20 minutes (Table 8.4).

More important, as shown in Figure 8.8, is that staff with counseling caseloads spent at least 50% of their time in face-to-face contact with their patients and another 17% of their time working directly in behalf of their patients.

Table 8.4   MMT Program Direct Care Staff's Caseloads and Counseling Sessions, by Position

			Counseling Sessions		
Position	**Active Caseload (%)**	**Active Monthly Cases (mean no.)**	**Individual (%)**	**Individual (mean no. min.)**	**Group (mean no. min.)**
Case manager	95.4	44.3	89.8	30.0	29.6
Counselor	99.0	40.3	85.4	36.3	45.9
Nurse	15.7	32.3	83.8	33.8	17.4
Clinical supervisor	85.6	23.5	82.2	39.6	48.3
Intake worker	47.6	29.5	86.7	40.6	12.7
Other	70.6	40.7	86.0	35.2	31.9

Figure 8.8   Time Distribution of MMT Direct Care Staff

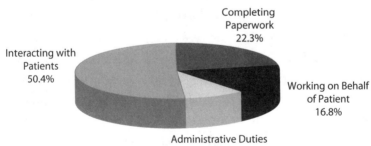

Completing Paperwork
22.3%

Interacting with Patients
50.4%

Working on Behalf of Patient
16.8%

Administrative Duties
9.6%

The study found that physicians tended to work part-time at MMT programs, 16 hours a week on average. Almost half of a physician's time was spent either conducting initial physical exams (26%) or reviewing patient dosing levels (20%; Figure 8.9). Physicians also reported in write-in categories that they spent time on other activities, such as treating emergencies, conducting psychiatric evaluations, performing initial medical care, and treating dual-diagnosis patients.

Physicians at larger MMT programs and those at programs in the largest urban areas spent a significantly smaller percentage of their time reviewing patient dosing. It is unknown what impact these practices had on service delivery and patient outcomes.

The ratio of physicians to patients was also evaluated per 100 patients by program type. Overall, there was approximately one full-time physician for every 400 patients. Ratios increased significantly as the size of the program decreased. Nonurban and large urban programs also had higher ratios than urban programs.

Figure 8.9   Time Distribution of MMT Physicians

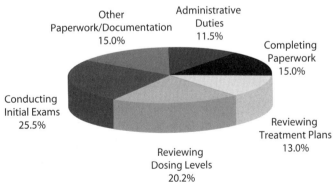

Other Paperwork/Documentation 15.0%

Administrative Duties 11.5%

Completing Paperwork 15.0%

Conducting Initial Exams 25.5%

Reviewing Treatment Plans 13.0%

Reviewing Dosing Levels 20.2%

ARE MMT PROGRAM STAFF ENCOURAGED TO ATTEND ONGOING TRAINING?

Providing MMT direct care staff with ongoing clinical training in a variety of areas is considered a best practice to encourage staff development and retention. Intake workers reported attending the most administrative trainings (an average of 5.3 in the past 6 months). Nurses reported attending the fewest (an average of 1.7 in the past 6 months; Figure 8.10).

Figure 8.10   Trainings Attended by MMT Direct Care Staff in the Past 6 Months, by Position

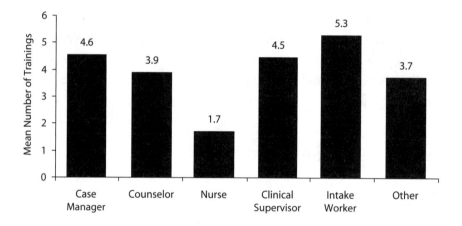

The number and types of trainings attended differed significantly across direct care staff positions. Clinical supervisors, intake workers, and counselors were most likely to attend all types of clinical trainings, except professional meetings or conferences. More than half of the case managers had obtained clinical training. In contrast, more than half of the nurses had attended professional meetings, and less than half had attended any other types of trainings.

Overall, direct care staff with a caseload had attended an average of four trainings in the past 6 months and 30 hours of training in the past year (Table 8.5). A larger percentage reported attending clinical trainings than administrative trainings.

**Table 8.5 Trainings Attended by MMT Direct Care Staff with a
Counseling Caseload, Past 6 Months**

Training Attended	Value
Trainings attended (mean no.)	4.0
Clinical seminars lasting 1–5 days (%)	62.3
Administrative trainings lasting 1–5 days (%)	22.1
Clinical seminars lasting less than 1 day (%)	59.4
Administrative seminars lasting less than 1 day (%)	26.8
Professional meetings or conferences (%)	61.9

WHAT IS THE RETENTION RATE AMONG MMT DIRECT CARE STAFF?

The Evaluation Study found that MMT programs were undergoing significant change. Staff turnover was noted as an issue in 18% of the sample, and about 40% reported a major change (e.g., new ownership, new site or site director, or new approaches to treatment) in the past 6 months. Staff retention is a critical aspect of providing high-quality treatment services. Unfortunately, MMT program staff are often underpaid (because of narrow program budgets and high costs of service delivery) and are not provided with developmental and support services associated with staff retention.

WHAT ARE THE PERCEPTIONS OF DIRECT CARE STAFF ABOUT TREATMENT SERVICES AND WORKING ENVIRONMENTS?

Staff perceptions of services are an important tool for assessing the quality of care. As such, the study surveyed staff regarding their perceptions of services offered through their MMT programs. Across labor categories, medical and psychological services were perceived by the largest percentage of direct care staff as fully adequate. The smallest percentage of direct care staff perceived assistance with housing/food and legal services as fully adequate (Table 8.6).

Direct care staff's perceptions of peer relationships and their working environments were generally positive. More than half direct care staff (54%) found their working relationships to be very supportive; however, there were differences across positions. Case managers and counselors were more likely than other staff to perceive working relationships as "very" or "somewhat" adversarial (16%). In contrast, the same was true for only 10% of intake workers.

As a place to work, the majority of direct care staff (59%) perceived their programs as "better than most"; however, there were significant differences across positions. More than three-quarters of clinical supervisors (76%) considered their organizations to be better than most; the same was true for just over half of the counselors (57%) and nurses (54%).

The study found significant differences by site location in physicians' perceptions of whether services were fully adequate. Physicians in large urban areas were more likely than their counterparts in less urban areas to find employment/education and family/social services to be fully adequate. Legal services, though rare, were more likely to be considered fully adequate by physicians at for-profit than at nonprofit or public programs.

Overall, more than two-thirds (69%) of physicians reported that the program they worked for was better than most. Physicians at for-profit programs were significantly more likely than physicians at nonprofit or public programs to report that their programs were better than most.

Table 8.6   MMT Direct Care Staff Who Perceived Services as Fully Adequate, by Position

	Service (%)						
	Employment/ Education	Family/ Social	Housing/ Food	Legal	Life Skills	Medical	Psych
Position							
Case manager	31.7	30.2	19.9	15.4	30.4	41.2	28.4
Counselor	28.9	30.5	20.7	14.8	29.5	52.6	48.3
Nurse	28.0	33.8	23.0	15.0	28.6	53.2	48.0
Clinical supervisor	26.7	24.9	18.5	20.5	36.3	50.0	50.1
Intake worker	8.6	45.5	8.6	0.0	15.9	33.6	58.1
Other	34.0	38.6	24.6	22.0	32.8	52.3	43.5

SUMMARY

- The Evaluation Study found that, as in many service delivery systems, there was an overrepresentation of White females among MMT staff. The proportion of African American and Hispanic direct care staff, however, was representative of the population as a whole.

- As expected, clinical supervisors were in the older age category. They also had more education and certifications than other staff groups. Half of the clinical supervisors surveyed held a graduate degree.

- The nursing staff, who are key to methadone dosing, generally had a low level of education. The majority of the nursing staff had an associate's degree or less education and were the least likely to have received additional training.

- MMT staff in recovery played a somewhat minor role in these programs; on average, they made up less than 20% of program staff.

- State certification was the most common type. Overall, however, less than half of the direct care staff had this certification, and almost half had no certification. Most who had certification were supervisors with more time in the system.

- As expected, MMT program staff were mainly full-time employees and spent most of their time interacting with patients. They spent the rest of their time on paperwork or efforts on behalf of clients. Physicians were usually part-time and split their time between direct medical care and indirect medical duties.

- Physicians represented a much more experienced group of staff. Although most program staff had attended a good number of trainings on average, the nurses with less education were the least likely to get training, possibly indicating an area needing skill enhancement.

- Relationships among staff and the environment were generally positive, but as expected for staff working with patients, case managers and counselors noted some adversarial relationships. Relationships were also strained when services were not adequately meeting patient needs.

- Physicians at for-profit MMT programs reported that ancillary services were more fully adequate in meeting patient needs. These physicians also reported more positively about their working environments.

CHAPTER 9—Methadone Maintenance Treatment Patients

Understanding patient characteristics is fundamental to understanding MMT. In this chapter, we describe the characteristics of patients receiving MMT services, starting with demographic characteristics and how they have changed over time. We review topics of special interest, including involvement with the criminal justice system, physical and psychological health, substance use, and services received.

WHO ARE THE PATIENTS RECEIVING MMT SERVICES?

The Evaluation Study found that over half of MMT patients were White males aged 35 or older (Table 9.1). A sizeable proportion of African Americans (23%) and Hispanics (25%) were also represented in the patient population, but there were relatively few patients of other races. The large proportion of patients identifying themselves as an "other" race (17%) may be explained by two factors: some patients may have identified more with a nationality than with a race, and many may have identified more with their multiracial heritage than with race as traditionally conceptualized. Half of the patients (50%) were employed for 35 or more hours a week.

HOW DO MMT PATIENTS TODAY COMPARE WITH PATIENTS FROM PREVIOUS NATIONAL STUDIES ON SUBSTANCE ABUSE TREATMENT?

The Evaluation Study findings on patient demographics are consistent with those of other large-scale studies assessing patients in substance abuse treatment. The finding that 42% of patients in MMT were female is similar to other study findings for the proportion of female patients: 43% in the California Drug and Alcohol Treatment Assessment (CALDATA; Gerstein et al., 1997), 39% in the Drug Abuse Treatment Outcomes Study (DATOS; Wechsberg, Craddock, & Hubbard, 1998), 32% in the National Treatment Improvement Evaluation Study (NTIES; DHHS, 1997), and 45% in the

Table 9.1   MMT Patient Demographics

	Percent
Gender	
Male	57.5
Age	
18–24	4.2
25–34	17.9
35–44	41.6
45–54	31.2
55 or older	5.2
Race	
African American	23.0
American Indian or Alaska Native	3.1
Asian or other Pacific Islander	1.4
Hispanic	24.6
White	55.6
Other	16.9
Working 35 or more hours a week	
Yes	50.5

Services Research Outcomes Study (SROS; SAMHSA, 1998). As shown in Table 9.2, the Evaluation Study found that 78% of patients were aged 35 or older. This finding is similar to the findings of other studies: SROS found that 72% were aged 35 or older, NTIES found that 83% were in this age range, and DATOS found that 43% of female patients and 63% of male patients were aged 36 or older. The 25% of Hispanics reported here compares with 12% in SROS and 25% in NTIES and DATOS. Racial composition across the studies is more difficult to compare because of the wide variability in the reported percentages. The Evaluation Study finding for proportion of White patients (56%) is closest to the finding in CALDATA (51%) and SROS (47%); NTIES reported 28%. For African American patients, NTIES and SROS reported 47% and 39%, respectively, compared with 48% reported in DATOS and 23% in the Evaluation Study. Comparable full-time employment data for the large-scale studies are not available.

Table 9.2 Demographic Variables of MMT Patients, by Study

	Study (%)				
	CALDATA	SROS	NTIES	DATOS	Evaluation
Gender and Age					
Female	43	45	32	40	43
Age 35+	91	72	83	82	78
Race					
African American non-Hispanic	5	39	47	48	23
African American or Hispanic	43	51	72	52	48
Hispanic	38	12	25	13	25
White non-Hispanic	51	47	28	39	56
Other	6	2			17

HOW DO THE GENERAL CHARACTERISTICS OF MMT PATIENTS DIFFER BY GENDER AND RACE?

Previous studies have identified important differences in the general demographic characteristics of MMT patients by gender and race. For example, females in MMT have more employment problems, such as higher unemployment rates at admission and lack of marketable skills (Craddock, Hubbard, Rachal, & Ginzburg, 1981; Marsh & Simpson, 1986). Males, on the other hand, enter MMT with more legal and financial problems (Craddock et al., 1981) and more criminal involvement (Kosten, Rounsaville, & Kleber, 1985; Rowan-Szal et al., 2000; Wechsberg et al., 1998).

Research has also begun to identify and address differential treatment needs by race. For example, Nurco, Hanlon, and Kinlock (1990) found that White males had the highest occupational status and level of education, compared with patients of other races.

Figures 9.1 and 9.2 show several demographic characteristics by race and gender using data from the Evaluation Study. Most of the MMT patient population was aged 35 or older (Figure 9.1). This was true of 92% of African

American males, 82% of African American females, 78% of White males, and 73% of White females.

Figure 9.1   African American and White Males and Females in MMT, by Age

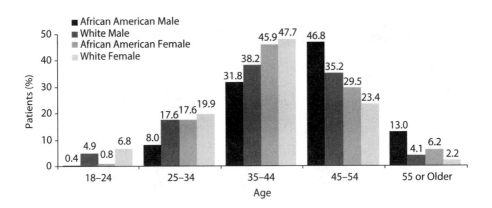

Overall, 28% of the patient population reported being ill, disabled, or unable to work. The rates were highest among African American males (32%), whereas African American females were least likely to report this condition (23%; Figure 9.2). Approximately one-fourth of both White males and females reported this condition (about 26% each). White males were most likely to report being employed full-time (61%); the same was true for less than half (42% to 47%) of the other race-gender groups.

HOW HAVE MMT PATIENT GENDER AND RACIAL CHARACTERISTICS CHANGED OVER THE PAST DECADE?

Although opiate dependence has traditionally been considered largely a male problem (Rowan Szal, Chatham, Joe, & Simpson, 2000), recent studies indicate that this is no longer the case. The number of females in treatment is not only large but is increasing. For example, data collected through the

Drug Abuse Reporting Program (DARP) between 1969 and 1971 showed that 22% of MMT patients were female (Curtis & Simpson, 1976). By the period between 1979 and 1981, the Treatment Outcome Prospective Study (TOPS) showed that 32% of patients were female (Chatham, Hiller, Rowan-Szal, Joe, & Simpson, 1999). Recent studies report figures on the percentage of female patients ranging up to 40% (Chatham et al., 1999; Chou, Hser, & Anglin, 1998; Magura, Nwakeze, Kang, & Demsky, 1999). Three other studies documenting substantial proportions of females in MMT include DATOS (39%), NTIES (32%), and SROS (45%; Wechsberg, Craddock, & Hubbard, 1998). Measured in 1999 to 2000, the Evaluation Study showed that 43% of MMT patients were female (Table 9.2).

African Americans comprise a greater percentage of the MMT patient population than of the general U.S. population (13%; U.S. Census Bureau, 2000). NTIES reported that 39% of MMT patients were African American, and SROS reported 47%. DATOS, however, reported that only 29% of male patients and 27% of female patients were African American. Although the Evaluation Study found that the majority of patients were White (56%), it found a proportion of African American patients (23%) similar to the proportion found in DATOS. About 17% of patients identified themselves as an "other" race (Table 9.2).

Figure 9.2   African American and White Males and Females in MMT, by Employment

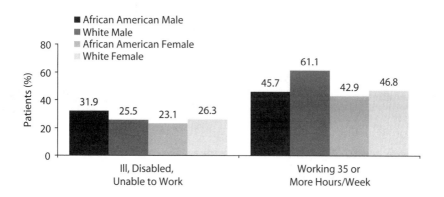

Across outpatient drug treatment programs (73% of which were MMTs), D'Aunno, Vaughn, and McElroy (1999) documented the changes in several patient and program characteristics from 1988 through 1995. This study, based on panel surveys of directors at 172 substance abuse treatment facilities within 116 MMT units, showed the percentage of African American patients rising from 27% in 1988 to 35% in 1995.

As a result of these patient population trends, the MMT system can expect to admit substantial and increasing numbers of females and African Americans over time. Because, as a group, male and female patients and those of different races have been found to have important differences in their behavioral characteristics and service needs, treatment providers and policy makers need to periodically reassess the demographic makeup of patient populations to ensure that the services provided are appropriate and effective.

HOW MANY MMT PATIENTS ARE INVOLVED WITH THE CRIMINAL JUSTICE SYSTEM?

There is a belief among the general public that the majority of patients in MMT are criminals or are involved with the criminal justice system. The Evaluation Study, as well as other studies, found that male patients were more likely than female patients to be involved with the criminal justice system and also more likely to become criminally involved earlier in their lives (Hser, Anglin, & Booth, 1987; Wechsberg, Cavanaugh, Dunteman, & Smith, 1994). The Evaluation Study findings show that about 20% of patients reported involvement to some extent with the criminal justice system. Most of these patients were on probation (about 12% of the total sample), and about 6% of patients were in required substance abuse treatment (treatment mandated by the judicial system). These findings are slightly lower than those reported in previous studies. For example, about 27% of patients in CALDATA and 29% in NTIES were involved with the criminal justice system (California Department of Alcohol and Drug Programs, 2004).

There were no significant differences by race or gender concerning patient-reported legal problems, except for awaiting charges or sentencing

(Figure 9.3). Of all the race-gender groups, African American females were least likely (2%) and White females were most likely (6%) to report that they were awaiting charges or sentencing.

Figure 9.3   African American and White Males and Females in MMT, by Legal Involvement

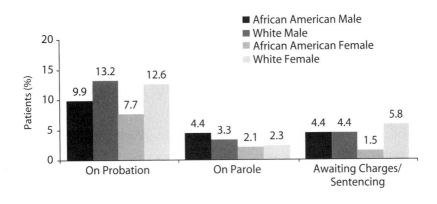

HOW LONG DO MMT PATIENTS STAY IN TREATMENT?

The CSAT *State Methadone Treatment Guidelines* state that patients should remain in MMT for as long as needed. The clinical decision on the length of time a patient should remain in MMT is a medical one, determined between the treatment physician and individual patient, with input from the entire interdisciplinary treatment team. MMT programs typically conduct annual assessments of patients to determine continued need for treatment.

The Evaluation Study findings shown in Figure 9.4 suggest that many patients remain in continuous MMT for more than 2 years (41%). Findings from this study also suggest that patients often seek MMT more than once. About 58% of patients in this study reported having received MMT previously.

Figure 9.4   Patient Continuous Time in MMT in Program

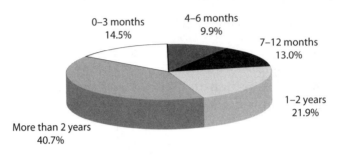

WHAT IS THE PHYSICAL HEALTH STATUS OF PATIENTS IN MMT?

Opiate users often experience extreme deterioration of health due to long-term drug use. Because opiates are often injected, users are at high risk for infectious diseases, including HIV/AIDS, HBV and HCV, and tuberculosis (CSAT, 2005).

Evaluation Study findings show that the majority of MMT patients reported their health as either good (32%) or very good (22%). About 10% of patients reported their health as poor, and 10% reported their health as excellent. The majority of patients (72%) reported having no health insurance.

WHAT IS THE PHYSICAL HEALTH STATUS OF PATIENTS IN MMT, BY GENDER AND RACE?

The Evaluation Study examined the physical health of patients over the 3-month period before they completed the survey. Because other studies have demonstrated the importance of reporting differences in health status by gender and race (Brown, Ajuluchukwu, Gonzalez, & Chu, 1992; Schiff, El-Bassel, Engstrom, & Gilbert, 2002), where possible the Evaluation Study data are displayed by gender or race. Findings show that females were less likely than males (29% versus 37%) to report their health status as excellent or very good (Figure 9.5).

Figure 9.5   Self-Reported Health Status of MMT Patients, by Gender

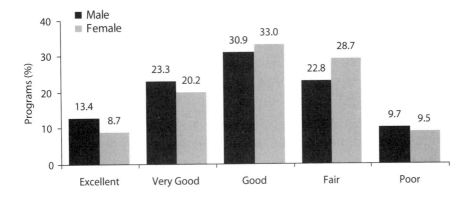

The Evaluation Study found that more males than females reported having health insurance (31% versus 25%). Males and females did not differ significantly in health-attributable difficulty performing regular activities during the 3 months before the survey (Table 9.3). African American males, however, did report having more difficulty performing daily activities because of physical health, compared with White males.

The Evaluation Survey also examined patients' need for hospitalization and number of visits to an emergency room in the past 3 months. As shown in Table 9.3, African American males and females reported using emergency room services at a slightly higher average rate than White males and females.

WHAT IS THE PSYCHOLOGICAL HEALTH STATUS OF PATIENTS IN MMT?

In addition to physical complications of opiate use, one study (Brooner, King, Kidorf, Schmidt, & Bigelow, 1997) found that nearly half of all patients in MMT had a co-occurring mental health disorder during their lifetime. Two representative studies found that patients in MMT had high occurrences of mood disorders, personality disorders, and anxiety disorders (Brooner et al., 1997; Mason et al., 1998). Several research studies have reported that females in MMT had higher rates of psychological and family problems than males (Craddock et al. 1981; Marsh & Simpson, 1986; Rowan-

Szal et al., 2000); more dependent children and related issues (Wechsberg et al., 1998); more violence issues, including more physical and sexual abuse (Wechsberg et al., 1998); and more HIV/AIDS-related issues and needs (Grella, Annon, & Anglin, 1996; Rowan-Szal et al., 2000).

The Evaluation Study findings show that 2% of MMT patients reported thinking about suicide "a little," 7% reported thinking about suicide "somewhat," and 5% reported thinking about suicide "a lot." About 13% of patients reported "quite a bit" of difficulty performing activities due to emotional health, and 4% could not perform daily activities at all because of emotional health.

Evaluators also asked patients about their feelings of stress/anxiety and depression. Patients were asked to respond to several questions (4 items on the stress/anxiety scale and 7 items on the depression scale) to which they were asked to respond using a 4-point scale ranging from 1 ("not at all") to 4 ("a lot"). Values of 1 to 4 were assigned to each response so that a mean score over the items could be calculated. Thus, a relatively low mean score over all items indicates a low likelihood of symptoms on that scale for that patient, and a relatively high mean score indicates a higher likelihood of symptoms. Overall, patients in MMT reported a mean score of 1.8 on the stress/anxiety scale and a mean score of 2.1 on the depression scale.

Table 9.3   Physical Health of African American and White Males and Females in MMT

	Patient			
	Male		Female	
	African American	White	African American	White
Physical Health				
Difficulty with daily activities because of physical health (*Some/quite a bit/could not do*)	37.6%	34.6%	36.7%	39.6%
Number of nights spent in hospital in past 3 months (mean)	1.0	0.8	0.5	0.7
Number of visits to ER in past 3 months (mean)	0.5	0.4	0.6	0.4

WHAT IS THE PSYCHOLOGICAL HEALTH STATUS OF PATIENTS IN MMT, BY GENDER AND RACE?

Patients were asked to report on their psychological health in the past 3 months. Males and females reported thinking about suicide in the past 3 months equally (24%). Females were significantly more likely than males, however, to report having difficulty performing regular activities because of emotional health (19% versus 15%). Among females, Whites reported a higher rate of difficulty with daily activities because of emotional health than African Americans (Table 9.4).

As shown in Table 9.4, White males and females, on average, had higher levels of both anxiety and depression than their gender or race counterparts. In addition, African American and White females reported higher levels of anxiety and depression, on average, compared with their male counterparts.

Table 9.4   Emotional Health of African American and White Males and Females in MMT

| | Patient | | | |
| | Male | | Female | |
	African American	White	African American	White
Emotional Health				
Difficulty with daily activities because of physical health (*Some/quite a bit/could not do*)	30.2%	32.0%	33.3%	38.5%
How much did you think about suicide? (*Somewhat/a lot*)	8.5%	11.5%	10.3%	11.3%
Mean score on anxiety scale (mean)	1.4	1.7	1.6	2.0
Mean score on depression scale (mean)	1.8	2.1	2.0	2.3

WHAT SUBSTANCES DO PATIENTS REPORT USING BEFORE AND DURING MMT?

Although MMT programs are generally effective in reducing the use of heroin and other opiates, previous research has shown that patients in these programs often continue to use other illicit drugs. Condelli, Dunteman, and Fairbank (1993) reported that drug testing results often show patients still using heroin, cocaine, tranquilizers, barbiturates, sedatives, marijuana, and alcohol. Although continued drug use among patients in MMT is not uncommon, a study using TOPS data found that patients dramatically reduced their use of heroin while in treatment (Hubbard et al., 1989). The same study also found that patient use of other drugs, including cocaine, sedatives, and alcohol, declined while patients were in MMT.

Table 9.5 presents the proportion of patients in the Evaluation Study who reported using alcohol, marijuana, crack or cocaine, and tranquilizers in the 3 months before the survey. These data show that there is considerable substance use among MMT patients. Alcohol was the substance used most often overall (about 32% reported some alcohol use in the past 3 months). Marijuana was the second most used substance (about 24% reported some use in the past 3 months). Self-reports indicate, however, that more patients used marijuana (5%) and tranquilizers (9%) daily than alcohol (4%).

Because of differing time frames and measuring instruments, it is difficult to compare, even generally, the findings of other large-scale studies with the findings presented here. For example, NTIES reported that 44% of pretreatment and 26% of follow-up MMT patients had used marijuana five times or more during the past year. DATOS reported that 89% of pretreatment and 28% of post-treatment MMT patients had used heroin once a week or more during the past year.

About 31% of respondents in the Evaluation Study reported some heroin use during the past 3 months, and about 5% reported daily use. This high percentage may be partly attributable to responses from patients who had been in treatment for less than the 3-month period specified in the question (about 15% of the patient population) and to responses from relatively new patients who had not yet stabilized on their methadone dosage. For these reasons, heroin use is examined by time in treatment (Figure 9.6).

Table 9.5   MMT Patient Frequency of Alcohol and Other Drug Use during the Past 3 Months

	Frequency of Use (%)					
	Daily	**3–6 Days a Week**	**1–2 Days a Week**	**1–3 Days a Month**	**Less Than Once a Month**	**Not at All**
Drug						
Alcohol	3.5	3.7	5.3	7.5	12.3	67.7
Marijuana	5.4	2.8	3.0	4.9	7.8	76.1
Cocaine or crack	1.9	2.4	3.2	4.9	8.5	79.2
Painkillers	4.1	2.2	2.1	4.9	7.5	79.3
Stimulants	0.9	0.4	0.6	1.3	2.2	94.6
Intravenous drugs	4.1	2.6	2.8	4.7	6.6	79.2
Tranquilizers	8.6	2.3	2.8	4.0	7.2	75.2

Figure 9.6   Proportion of MMT Patients Reporting Heroin Use During the Past 3 Months, by Time in Treatment

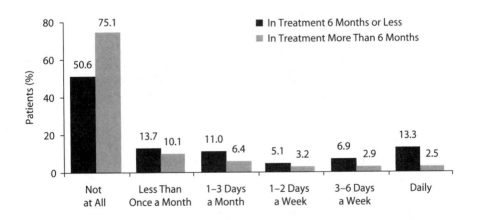

There is a strong association between time in treatment and heroin use; patients in treatment for more than 6 months use heroin less. This relationship could be explained by the interplay of factors other than the positive impact of treatment. For example, patients in treatment for longer periods may be more stable in their recovery; that is, patients who continue to use heroin after beginning treatment may be discharged from treatment by MMT programs that have low- or zero-tolerance policies for nonabstinent behavior. Further, patients who continue to use heroin after entering treatment may not be ready to deal with their addictions and may voluntarily withdraw. For patients remaining in treatment for more than 6 months, however, a significant difference in heroin use (specifically, daily use versus abstinence) is seen in self-reports. About 13% of patients in treatment for less than 6 months reported daily heroin use, versus only 3% of patients in treatment for 6 months or more. Additionally, 75% of patients in treatment for 6 months or more reported no heroin use, versus only 51% of patients in treatment for less than 6 months.

HOW DOES SUBSTANCE USE BY MMT PATIENTS DIFFER BY GENDER AND RACE?

Males and females in MMT have reported different substance use patterns. For example, males entering MMT have been found to have more severe alcohol-related problems than females (Rowan-Szal et al., 2000; Wechsberg et al., 1998). The Evaluation Study examined substance use during the past 3 months and found differences by gender and race (Table 9.6). In relation to alcohol, African American and White females were more likely to be nonusers than males in their respective racial group. Of the four groups, African American males were most likely to use alcohol (40%). Fewer respondents overall reported using marijuana than alcohol. As with alcohol, females were less likely to have used marijuana than males in their respective racial group. African American patients were less likely to have used marijuana than White patients. White males were most likely to have used marijuana (30%).

Racial differences were apparent for use of other drugs as well. White patients were less likely to have used cocaine or heroin, and African American patients were less likely to have used tranquilizers or a needle. Within each racial group, there were less pronounced differences by gender.

Table 9.6   Substance Use During the Past 3 Months Among African American and White Males and Females in MMT

	Patient (%)			
	Male		Female	
	African American	White	African American	White
Alcohol				
Not at all	59.8	65.7	69.2	74.1
Monthly	21.5	20.5	16.1	18.6
Weekly	15.2	9.6	11.0	5.6
Daily	3.4	4.3	3.7	1.8
Marijuana				
Not at all	79.4	69.8	83.1	76.9
Monthly	13.0	14.8	12.9	12.0
Weekly	3.9	6.9	3.1	6.7
Daily	3.2	8.5	1.0	4.4
Cocaine				
Not at all	70.1	83.6	67.4	81.6
Monthly	18.2	10.8	19.2	12.9
Weekly	8.8	4.7	9.3	4.3
Daily	2.8	1.0	4.2	1.3
Heroin				
Not at all	61.8	70.1	66.6	72.9
Monthly	23.9	15.2	19.4	15.9
Weekly	8.4	8.2	6.8	7.2
Daily	5.9	4.5	7.2	4.0
Tranquilizers				
Not at all	88.9	70.7	88.0	66.5
Monthly	6.2	13.3	7.7	13.9
Weekly	2.6	6.2	2.3	5.4
Daily	2.3	10.4	2.0	14.2
Use of Needle				
Not at all	81.2	76.3	85.4	77.0
Monthly	10.4	12.2	8.2	13.2
Weekly	4.9	6.8	2.9	5.6
Daily	3.6	4.6	3.5	4.3

WHAT TREATMENT SERVICES DO MMT PATIENTS REPORT RECEIVING?

In addition to providing methadone dosing to patients, MMT programs offer a variety of ancillary treatment services, including individual and group counseling, educational services, and medical care. Numerous studies have found that programs that offer ancillary services to patients report better outcomes than programs providing few or no ancillary services (Kidorf, King, & Brooner, 1999; Magura et al., 1999).

Figure 9.7 shows the proportion of patients receiving core and ancillary services during the past 3 months. According to Evaluation Study data, patients more often received individual counseling (78%) than group counseling (43%). This finding is in contrast to the findings of other studies, which have shown group counseling to be an effective and economical alternative to individual counseling under certain circumstances.

Figure 9.7   Proportion of MMT Patients Receiving Core and Ancillary Services in the Past 3 Months

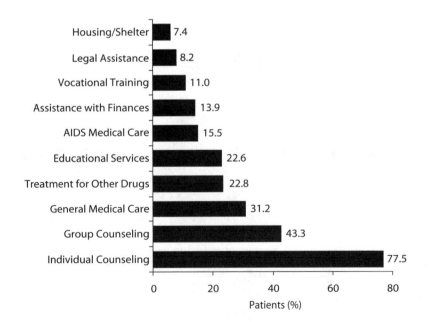

Note. Because multiple responses were allowed, percentages do not sum to 100.

The findings also indicate that nearly 23% of patients received treatment for use of substances other than opiates. This statistic highlights the problem of polysubstance use among the MMT patient population and emphasizes the need for more comprehensive treatment to address heroin and other substance abuse or dependence.

Long-term use of opiates and other drugs, including alcohol, has been shown to negatively affect health status; access to ongoing medical care is therefore an important component of high-quality services. The finding that only 31% of patients reported receiving any general medical care in the past 3 months indicates that this need is not being addressed.

HOW DO TREATMENT SERVICES RECEIVED DIFFER BY GENDER AND RACE?

Because of the variation in treatment service needs by gender and race, it is important to consider whether treatment services received differ along the same dimensions. Among the most successful substance abuse interventions and treatments are ones that strive to be culturally sensitive with respect to patients' race; that is, they account for how patients' different cultural experiences result in different needs for specific types of treatment. For example, health services research suggests that the race of a patient relative to the race of the attending clinic personnel is an important factor in the patient's level of comfort, comprehension of the treatment regimen, trust in interacting with clinic personnel, and subsequent outcomes (Cooper-Patrick et al., 1999). Saha et al. (2000) also found that patients often prefer and seek out physicians whose race is similar to their own, and Gray and Stoddard (1997) reported that minority patients were five times more likely than nonminorities to have a minority general physician.

The Evaluation Study found no significant differences by race or gender in the proportions of patients who reported receiving individual counseling. However, a higher percentage of African American than White males and females reported receiving group counseling (Figure 9.8).

African American patients were more likely than White patients to have received a variety of support services, including educational, vocational, and legal assistance (Figure 9.9). A similar pattern was not found by gender.

African American males and females were more likely than White males and females to report receiving AIDS-related services and treatment services for dependence on or abuse of nonopiates (Figure 9.10). White males and females were equally likely to receive these two services, whereas African American males were more likely than African American females to have received AIDS-related medical care, and African American females were more likely to have received treatment for abuse of substances other than opiates. A higher percentage of White females than White males reported receiving general medical care, whereas the opposite was true among African American males and females.

Figure 9.8   African American and White Males and Females in MMT Receiving Individual and Group Counseling

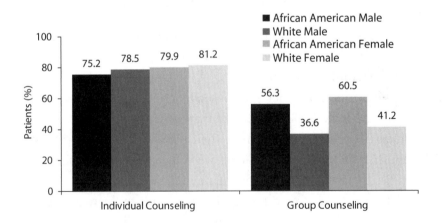

Figure 9.9   African American and White Males and Females in Treatment Receiving Educational, Vocational, or Legal Services

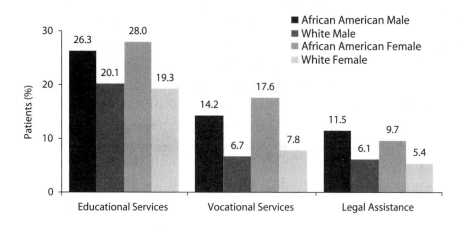

Figure 9.10   African American and White Males and Females in MMT Receiving Medical Care or Treatment for Dependence on or Abuse of Nonopiates

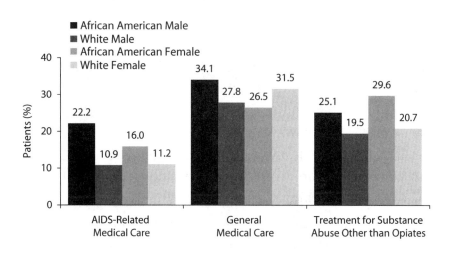

DO PATIENTS REPORT BEING SATISFIED WITH MMT SERVICES?

The Evaluation Study asked patients about their satisfaction with the MMT services they were receiving. Although estimates indicate that roughly half of the patients felt that they were never/rarely or sometimes involved in treatment decisions, about 61% of patients indicated that they were treated fairly most or all of the time by MMT staff. An even larger majority (83%) reported that they would not be afraid to file a formal grievance if they were treated unfairly. This generally positive attitude toward MMT programs and staff is summarized in the patients' overall satisfaction with treatment. Only 5% of patients rated their treatment as poor, whereas 33% rated their treatment as excellent.

Patient satisfaction varied somewhat by type of MMT program. For-profit programs were associated with higher reported patient involvement (34% versus 29%) and with higher treatment satisfaction (37% versus 29%) than their nonprofit or public counterparts. Additionally, patients at smaller programs reported greater involvement in treatment decisions than patients at large programs (36% versus 30%). Patients at smaller programs were also significantly more satisfied with treatment than patients at larger programs (43% versus 30% rating treatment as excellent).

SUMMARY

- The Evaluation Study and other large-scale studies have shown the MMT patient population to be diverse; that is, patients were not overwhelmingly of any specific gender, race, age, or employment status. However, patients appear to be aging, and treatment issues may therefore change.
- African American patients (especially males) tended to be older than their White counterparts, and White female patients tended to be younger than other demographic groups.
- African American male patients were most likely to report being ill, disabled, or unable to work, relative to the other groups.
- White male patients were most likely to report being employed full-time, relative to other racial and gender groups.

- White female patients reported the greatest difficulty with daily activities. White male and African American female patients reported a similar degree of difficulty.

- African American and White female patients reported higher mean scores for both anxiety and depression, compared with their male counterparts.

- Many MMT patients used substances while in treatment. Alcohol was the substance used most often overall, and marijuana was the second most used substance.

- African American patients were more likely than White patients to be recent cocaine and needle users.

- White patients were more likely to be recent heroin and tranquilizer users.

- A higher percentage of African American patients than White patients received group counseling, AIDS-related medical care, treatment for abuse of substances other than opiates, and educational, vocational, and legal support services.

CHAPTER 10—Accreditation Outcomes

MMT programs in the United States have been subject to accreditation since 2001. In this chapter, we explore the reasons for the regulatory shift to accreditation and detail the dimensions that accreditation standards address. We then explore accreditation outcomes, focusing on the areas in which MMT programs are doing well and those that need improvement. The chapter concludes with a discussion of the costs of achieving accreditation.

WHY WAS ACCREDITATION RECOMMENDED FOR MMT?

MMT continues to evolve, and advances in opiate dependence treatment research have greatly reduced the need to further study the effectiveness of MMT (Rettig & Yarmolinsky, 1995). Substance abuse treatment processes have been superseded by a focus on treatment outcomes. Thus, performance measurement, quality assurance, and accountability have become critical factors in monitoring substance abuse services.

Recently, because of increasing treatment demand and regulatory practice, policy makers established standard guidelines for use in the development of all standards to address outdated compliance regulations. In January 2001, Congress released new federal standards to improve the quality and clinical outcomes of MMT programs. These regulations are, in part, a response to GAO findings that the existing regulations for MMT did not ensure quality of care. Under the new regulations, oversight of MMT programs shifted from an FDA inspection model to a SAMHSA oversight administered accreditation model that implants working standards into the service delivery system nationwide to standardize care and provide MMT programs with the tools to govern themselves. These changes bring a new focus to the regulation and service delivery of opiate dependence treatment: performance and outcomes.

Historically, monitoring performance measurement standards has been the responsibility of various private-sector professional trade groups and associations. Much of the responsibility of performance measurement in the health care and rehabilitation arena has been passed to accreditation organizations, such as the Commission on Accreditation of Rehabilitation Facilities (CARF) and the Joint Commission on Accreditation of Healthcare Organizations (JCAHO). For example, the Centers for Medicare and Medicaid Services (CMS) relies on accreditation to certify approximately 7,000 hospitals that provide services to Medicare patients, and the Clinical Laboratory Improvement Act (CLIA) of 1998 uses private accreditation as the primary basis for certifying human clinical laboratories (DHHS, 1999). Additionally, several states now mandate accreditation across their public health care organizations (e.g., Michigan, Indiana, and North Carolina).

With accreditation organizations entrenched in performance measurement and outcome data collection, an accreditation-based system seemed a natural substitute for the process-oriented regulatory system used to monitor MMT. The Narcotic Drugs in Maintenance and Detoxification Treatment of Narcotic Dependence: Repeal of Current Regulations and Proposal to Adopt New Regulations, Proposed Rule (DHHS, 1999), and the Opioid Drugs in Maintenance and Detoxification Treatment of Opiate Addiction, Final Rule (DHHS, 2001), emphasized that an accreditation-based system would allow greater administrative flexibility, fewer constraints on clinical judgment, and more focus on the individual needs of patients.

Therefore, achieving accreditation through a CSAT-approved accrediting body is intended to prove that an MMT program has committed resources to ensure compliance with prescribed practices, including formal documentation activities; QA activities; continual evaluation of MMT program practices, procedures, and outcomes; and continual evaluation of patient care and outcomes. These practices are hypothesized to significantly predict positive patient outcomes. In other words, not only will accredited organizations be more effective than nonaccredited organizations, but the more an organization conforms to each of the accreditation standards, the more effective it will be (McCaughrin, 1991).

In addition to increasing effectiveness, national accreditation for MMT programs will increase standardization of care. Accreditation provides organizations with legitimacy, showing that they have adopted practices and structures accepted as appropriate by professional groups, thus increasing standardization of care across boundaries.

WHAT DOES ACCREDITATION ASSESS?

Private accreditation is a form of quality oversight. Under an accreditation-based system, organizations plan, organize, and run their programs in concert with a published set of standards. Programs then apply for review against these standards; if they conform sufficiently, they are awarded an accreditation certificate (Wilkerson, Migas, & Slaven, 2000). To ensure that services and supports are being effectively monitored, evaluated, and held to high performance standards, national accreditation bodies share many common principles and approaches.

To fulfill their accountability mission, MMT program accreditors must be adaptable and responsive to the changing environment. Accrediting bodies are themselves engaged in a competitive environment. Their performance is scrutinized, and if they fail to deliver high-quality services or keep current with developments, they lose customers and market share. To stay current, competitive, and responsive, accreditors must work collaboratively with professionals in the field to consistently apply science-based evidence to treatment service delivery. This approach of applying a science-to-service model was used to develop the CSAT guidelines that serve as the foundation for accreditation standards.

Specifically, the CSAT guidelines address a number of domains that are representative of the domains found in the Final Rule and serve to drive the development and revision of accreditation standards (CSAT, 2001). These domains are as follows:

- administrative organization and responsibilities
- management of facility and clinical environment
- risk management and continuous quality improvement
- professional staff credentials and development
- patient admission criteria

- patient medical and psychosocial assessment

- guidelines for therapeutic dosage

- treatment planning, evaluation of patient progress in treatment, and continuous clinical assessment

- testing for drug use

- unsupervised approved use (i.e., take-home medication)

- withdrawal and discharge

- management of concurrent alcohol and polysubstance abuse

- concurrent services

- special considerations

- care of women in treatment

- patient rights

- record keeping and documentation

- community relations and education

- diversion control

Using these treatment domains and guidelines, individual accreditation organizations can independently develop and incorporate methadone-specific accreditation standards into their behavioral health care standards, resulting in a comprehensive accreditation manual for MMT.

WHAT ARE THE POSSIBLE ACCREDITATION OUTCOMES?

Accreditation outcomes are specific to the individual accrediting body and vary by specific accreditation organization. CARF and JCAHO are two of the more prominent accreditation organizations in substance abuse treatment. Although these two organizations are similar in many aspects, they differ somewhat in their accreditation outcomes. CARF accreditation outcomes include the following (CARF, 1998):

- 3-year accreditation: The organization met the accreditation principles and conditions and showed substantial fulfillment of the standards.

- 1-year accreditation: The organization met each of the accreditation principles and conditions. Although there were deficiencies in relation to standards, there was evidence of the organization's capability, commitment to correcting the deficiencies, and progress toward their correction.

- Provisional accreditation: Following the expiration of a 1-year accreditation, a provisional accreditation is awarded to an organization that is still functioning at the same level as when originally accredited. A provisional accreditation is awarded for the period of a year, with the condition that the organization performs at the level of a 3-year accreditation on the next survey.

- Nonaccreditation: The organization had major deficiencies in several areas of the standards, and there were serious questions about its rehabilitative benefits and the health, welfare, or safety of its patients; the organization had failed over time to bring itself into substantial conformance with the standards, or it had failed to meet any one or more of the accreditation principles or conditions.

As part of its customary practice, CARF provides accreditation to the entire collection of behavioral health services within an organization.

JCAHO accreditation outcomes include the following (JCAHO, 2000):

- 3-year accreditation with full standard compliance (formerly accreditation with commendation): The organization demonstrated satisfactory compliance with applicable JCAHO standards in all performance areas.

- 3-year accreditation with requirements for improvement (formerly accreditation with type I recommendations): The organization demonstrated satisfactory compliance with applicable JCAHO standards in most performance areas but had deficiencies in one or more performance areas or in meeting accreditation policy requirements.

- Conditional accreditation: The organization failed to demonstrate compliance with applicable JCAHO standards in multiple performance areas, or it was persistently unable or unwilling to demonstrate satisfactory compliance with one or more JCAHO standards, or it failed to comply with one or more specified accreditation policy requirements but was believed to be capable of achieving acceptable compliance within a stipulated period. Upon review, this outcome could be converted to a 3-year accreditation outcome.

- Preliminary denial of accreditation: The organization failed to demonstrate satisfactory compliance with applicable JCAHO standards in multiple performance areas, or with accreditation policy requirements, or for other reasons. This accreditation decision is subject to subsequent review.

- Accreditation denied.

Other accreditation organizations (e.g., the Council on Accreditation [CAO]) have similar accreditation outcome categories.

WERE MMT PROGRAMS ACCREDITED BEFORE BEING REQUIRED TO SEEK ACCREDITATION UNDER THE NEW REGULATIONS?

Before the federal regulation requiring MMT programs to become accredited, several states encouraged accreditation of outpatient substance abuse treatment programs through the promotion of deemed status (Chriqui et al., 2006). Deemed status refers to state acceptance of accreditation in lieu of mandated licensure requirements. For example, MMT programs accredited by a recognized accreditation organization (e.g., CARF, JCAHO) are deemed under state law to be compliant with state licensure requirements. In a recent study, Chriqui et al. found that 49% of all states offered deemed status of some type to their outpatient treatment programs. Of these, 33% offered deemed status for JCAHO accreditation and 29% offered deemed status for CARF accreditation. Within the Evaluation Study, 22% of all programs reported being previously accredited by either JCAHO or CARF.

During the course of the Evaluation Study, 110 MMT programs received an accreditation outcome from either JCAHO or CARF (Table 10.1).

Table 10.1   MMT Program Accreditation Results

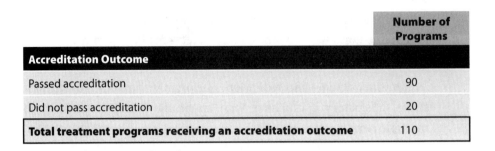

Accreditation Outcome	Number of Programs
Passed accreditation	90
Did not pass accreditation	20
Total treatment programs receiving an accreditation outcome	110

IN WHAT AREAS ARE MMT PROGRAMS PERFORMING WELL OR NEEDING IMPROVEMENT?

To assess the performance of MMT programs within specific treatment service categories, evaluators conducted an analysis of specific accreditation standard citations/recommendations received by an MMT program during the initial accreditation site visit in the Evaluation Study. This analysis focused on compliance with CARF accreditation standards. If an MMT program was not in compliance with an accreditation standard, it received a recommendation (Wechsberg et al., 2003) from the accrediting organization (CARF) noting the specific area of noncompliance. The total n for the analyses of accreditation standard recommendations is 68.

Nonprofit or public MMT programs received a greater number of recommendations in the areas of organizational quality, patient rights, and health and safety (Figure 10.1). For-profit programs received a greater number of recommendations in the areas of organizational administration, services, organizational planning, performance improvement, continuum of care, treatment planning, screening and assessment, and medication use. Overall, MMT programs reported the most difficulty with organizational administration, performance improvement, and screening and assessment. These findings support other Evaluation Study findings indicating that (1) there is little consistency across MMT programs in regard to patient screening and assessment, and (2) few programs have implemented a QA or continuous quality improvement plan.

Figure 10.1   Mean Total Accreditation Standard Citations Received, by Ownership

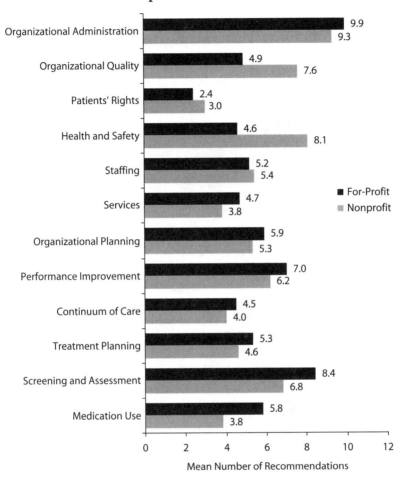

Figure 10.2 presents the mean total accreditation standard recommendations by MMT program size. Small programs received the greatest number of recommendations in the areas of organizational administration, services, organizational planning, performance improvement, continuum of care, screening and assessment, and medication use. Midsize programs received the greatest number of recommendations in the areas of patient rights and staffing. Large programs received the greatest number of recommendations in the areas of organizational quality and health and safety. Similar to

Figure 10.2   Mean Total Accreditation Standard Citations Received, by MMT Program Size

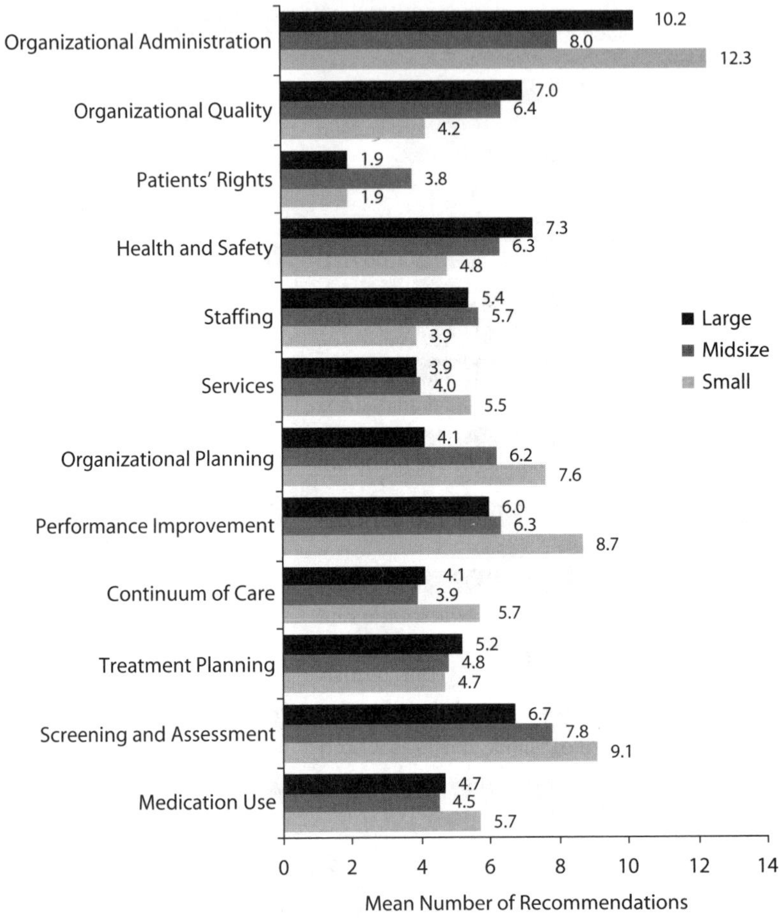

Note. Because of rounding, percentages may not sum to 100; Small = 0–100 patients; midsize = 101–300 patients; large = 301 or more patients.

findings on ownership above, overall, MMT programs reported the most difficulty with organizational administrative standards, performance improvement, and screening and assessment.

Figure 10.3 presents the mean total accreditation standard recommendations in nonurban, urban, and large urban MMT treatment programs. Nonurban programs received the greatest number of recommendations in the areas of patient rights, organizational planning, performance improvement, continuum of care, and medication use. Urban programs received the greatest number of recommendations in the areas of organizational quality, health and safety, staffing, services, treatment planning, and screening and assessment. Large urban programs received the greatest number of recommendations in the area of organizational administration. MMT programs again reported the most difficulty with the domains of organizational administration, performance improvement, and screening and assessment. Additionally, the organizational planning domain caused some difficulty within nonurban programs, as did the health and safety domain within urban programs.

Figure 10.3 Total Accreditation Standard Recommendations Received, by Urbanicity

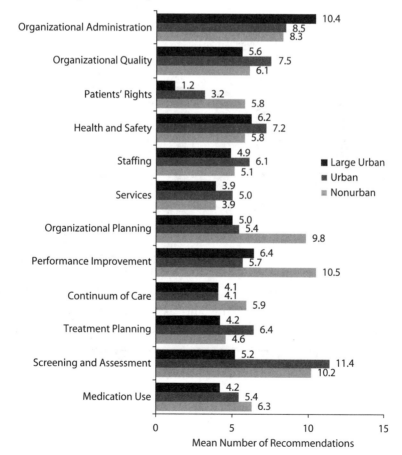

Over 80% of the eligible MMT programs in the Evaluation Study achieved accreditation from their initial accreditation survey. An analysis of accredited versus nonaccredited outcomes found no differential accreditation outcome by MMT program size, ownership, or urbanicity. However, an analysis of standard recommendations cited during the initial accreditation survey indicated that ownership was predictive of the amount of both methadone-related and general recommendations received by MMT programs (Figure 10.4). For-profit programs received fewer recommendations of either type during their accreditation surveys.

Figure 10.4   Total Methadone-Specific and General Accreditation Standard Recommendations Received, by Ownership, Size, and Urbanicity

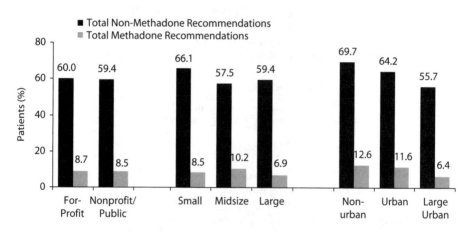

Overall, MMT programs experienced the most difficulty with the accreditation standard domains of organizational administration, performance measurement, and screening and assessment. Additionally, small nonurban and urban programs experienced the most difficulty, receiving the greatest number of total accreditation standard recommendations.

WHAT IS THE COST TO MMT PROGRAMS OF PURSUING ACCREDITATION?

The accreditation process involves months of preparation by program staff to comply with accreditation standards, followed by a survey visit from an external review body. Experience indicates that the months of preparation may consume the majority of resources the program spends in the accreditation process. Little research exists on the costs of accreditation in any field; with accreditation being new to the MMT field, there is virtually no information available on the cost to MMT programs of pursuing accreditation.

The Evaluation Study marked the first time that a systematic economic approach was applied to evaluating the costs and activities associated with pursuing accreditation in any field. As a result, the Evaluation Study provided a unique opportunity to evaluate the process of pursuing accreditation and to estimate the total economic costs to MMT programs associated with pursuing accreditation.

MMT programs engaged in eight primary activities to prepare for the accreditation survey, including staff meetings and training, as well as reviewing and updating the following: policies and procedures, record keeping, treatment plans and continuing care plans, admission procedures, storage of controlled substances, and facilities. An "other" category was included to capture any resources used in activities outside these eight activities.

To collect data on the time spent performing these activities and their associated nonlabor expenses, a survey instrument called the Accreditation Activity Log (AAL) was developed. Program staff used the AAL to collect data on the labor hours spent by staff on accreditation activities and expenditures on nonlabor resources (e.g., supplies, materials, and capital improvements) required for accreditation. The data on labor hours were collected by job type (e.g., counselor, nurse) and by activity (e.g., staff meetings, policy revisions, and facility renovation). The nonlabor resources data were collected by type of expenditure (e.g., facility, supplies, equipment or other capital, and other resources) and by activity. Following the Evaluation Study baseline site visit, program staff completed AALs every 2 weeks during the period of preparation for the accreditation survey visit and in the weeks following the visit as the program prepared its quality improvement report.

Table 10.2 presents mean total and per-patient cost estimates for pursuing accreditation, as well as the breakdown of costs into program preparation, technical assistance, and accreditation survey fees. The average cost of pursuing accreditation was $48,005 ($289 per patient); the majority of this cost was due to program preparation ($39,484). About 99% of the sites reported some type of program preparation activity. Technical assistance ($3,047) accounted for about 6% of the total costs. About 91% of the programs in the Evaluation Study received some type of technical assistance. Accreditation survey fees ($5,474) accounted for about 11% of the total costs of pursuing accreditation.

Table 10.2   Total and Per-Patient Costs of Pursuing Accreditation (2000$)

	Average Cost	
	Total	**Total per Patient**
Total cost, n=102[a]	$48,005	$289
Cost Breakdown		
Program preparation[b]	$39,484	$231
Technical assistance	$3,047	$20
Accreditation survey fees[c]	$5,474	$38

Source: Zarkin, Dunlap, & Homsi, 2006.

[a] Excludes programs that dropped out of the Evaluation Study before the follow-up visit, programs that did not undergo their accreditation survey during the study time frame, two cost outlier programs, and one program from the original sample that was excluded because the study's quality control review indicated that it was not an independent outpatient program as initially reported.

[b] Includes program labor and nonlabor costs incurred by the MMT program during accreditation preparation, plus the program's labor and nonlabor costs for initial trainings.

[c] Includes application and survey fees.

The mean estimates for total program preparation costs, labor preparation costs, and nonlabor preparation costs by preparation activity are provided in Table 10.3. The review and updating of policy and procedures accounted for the majority of the costs to pursue accreditation (approximately 22%), followed by staff meetings and training (approximately 17% each). The review and updating of the storage of controlled substances (approximately 2%), followed by the review and updating of admission procedures (approximately 4%), accounted for the smallest portions of total program preparation costs. Additionally, the majority of program preparation costs were due to labor hours. Labor costs accounted for approximately 83% of the total program preparation costs. Although some nonlabor costs were incurred in each activity, the majority of these costs were incurred in the review and upgrading of facilities ($3,476).

Table 10.3 Average Program Preparation Costs for Accreditation (2000$), by Activity, n=102

	Cost			
	Total Preparation	**Percentage of Total**	**Labor**	**Nonlabor**
Total	$39,484	100	$32,872	$6,612
Accreditation Preparation Activity				
Staff meeting	$6,634	17	$6,490	$145
Training	$6,408	16	$4,554	$1,854
Review/update policies and procedures	$8,596	22	$8,390	$207
Review/update records	$4,625	12	$4,363	$262
Review/update treatment plans	$4,094	10	$4,034	$60
Review/update admission procedures	$1,434	4	$1,397	$38
Review/update storage of controlled substances	$886	2	$702	$184
Review/update facilities	$5,156	13	$1,680	$3,476
Other	$1,649	4	$1,263	$387

Source: Zarkin et al., 2006.

HOW MANY STAFF HOURS ARE NEEDED TO PREPARE FOR ACCREDITATION?

Table 10.4 presents mean estimates of labor hours spent preparing for accreditation by activity. Programs in the Evaluation Study spent an average of 1,378 labor hours preparing for accreditation. The majority of staff time was spent reviewing and updating policies and procedures, which accounted for about 25% of the total program preparation time. Staff meetings accounted for about 20% of the total program preparation time. Program staff spent the least amount of time reviewing and updating storage procedures for controlled substances (2%).

Table 10.4   Average Site Preparation Hours by Activity, n=102

	Hours	
	Labor	**Percentage of Total**
Total	1,378	100
Accreditation Preparation Activity		
Staff meeting	271	20
Training	195	14
Review/update policies and procedures	340	25
Review/update records keeping	200	15
Review/update treatment plans	169	12
Review/update admission procedures	57	4
Review/update storage of controlled substances	28	2
Review/update facilities	63	5
Other	56	4

Source: Zarkin et al., 2006.

Mean estimates were calculated for the proportion of time program staff spent preparing for accreditation by job type. Staff job types were divided into eight categories:

- psychiatrists/physicians
- nurses (registered nurses, other licensed nurses)
- other medical staff (pharmacists, other medical personnel)
- counseling staff (psychologists, counselors)
- case management staff (case managers, social workers)
- other direct care staff (other therapists or rehabilitation specialists, teachers)
- administrative staff (program administrators, program supervisor/director, clerical)
- other staff (child care workers)

As shown in Table 10.5, administrative staff incurred the greatest burden in preparing for accreditation, accounting for almost 50% of the total hours spent. Counseling staff accounted for 21% of the total time spent in preparing for accreditation. Medical personnel (i.e., psychiatrists/physicians, nurses, other medical staff) accounted for about 17% of the total time, and most of this time was spent by nurses (12%).

Table 10.5 Average Proportion of Program Preparation Hours for Accreditation, by Job Type, n=102

Job Type	Average Proportion of Total Preparation Hours
Psychiatrists/physicians	0.04
Nurses	0.12
Other medical staff	0.01
Counseling staff	0.21
Case management staff	0.07
Other direct care staff	0.01
Administrative staff	0.49
Other staff	0.05

Source: Zarkin et al., 2006.

SUMMARY

- The majority of MMT programs will pass accreditation; however, most will do so with modifications to current policies and procedures.

- There is no evidence to suggest differential outcomes for small or rural programs.

- In general, the recommendations are concentrated in the domains of organizational administration, performance improvement, and screening and assessment.

- The average cost of pursuing accreditation was $48,005 ($289 per patient); the majority of this cost was due to program preparation ($39,484).

CHAPTER 11—Regulation of Methadone Maintenance Treatment

In the United States, MMT programs operate within a complex regulatory structure. Federal regulations provide universal rules for licensing and operation of MMT programs. State governments have separate regulatory authority, which they exert through policy, legislation, and funding. In addition, MMT programs may be subject to local regulations through zoning laws or other requirements. This chapter addresses each level of MMT regulation.

HOW DOES THE FEDERAL GOVERNMENT REGULATE MMT?

Three primary federal agencies are charged with the oversight and regulation of MMT:

- DEA is responsible for monitoring methadone distribution and preventing diversion.

- FDA is responsible for ensuring the safety and effectiveness of pharmacologic treatment.

- SAMHSA is responsible for determining standards for MMT and overseeing implementation and maintenance of those standards.

See Chapter 2 for a summary of the history of MMT regulation in the United States.

HOW DO STATES REGULATE MMT?

FDA regulations require each state to establish a state methadone authority (SMA) to oversee MMT within its jurisdiction. The bureaucratic entity responsible for overseeing MMT programs varies by state; in some states, multiple entities have oversight authority. The source of states' legal authority to regulate MMT may be statutory, regulatory, administrative, policy based, or some combination of these.

The Evaluation Study case study analysis of how five states approach regulation and oversight of MMT programs found that more than one agency had oversight authority in each state. In some states, separate government entities oversaw three functions: licensing, oversight, and diversion prevention. In some states, licensure (including applications for new programs) was separate from ongoing oversight; in others, these two functions were performed by the SMA. Several states had a separate agency overseeing controlled substances (paralleling DEA).

WHAT DO STATES REGULATE?

State regulations can be categorized according to eight domains, each of which includes a number of constructs (Table 11.1).

A 1999 analysis of MMT regulations in 14 states compared state regulations with FDA and DEA regulations governing MMT programs to identify the extent to which they were similar to or above the minimum federal MMT requirements. This analysis found that many states used significant aspects of the federal regulations as the core requirements for their state regulations. All study states had regulatory provisions different from or in addition to the federal regulatory provisions. The number of additional provisions ranged from 8 to 16 (Ameen, Sullivan, Malhotra, Ringel, & Harwood, 1999).

HOW DO STATES VARY IN THEIR REGULATION OF MMT?

The review and analysis of state regulations governing MMT programs showed that states varied considerably in their approaches to oversight, as evidenced by whether states specifically addressed the eight regulatory domains listed above (Roussel, Layton, & Squire, 2002).

To develop a framework for classifying states in terms of their regulatory approaches and to determine whether there were substantial similarities in these approaches, it was necessary to first identify the most significant regulatory dimensions. Using an evaluation of state documentation, five key dimensions were identified for MMT regulation:

Table 11.1 Categorization of State Regulations

Domain	Constructs
Roles and responsibilities of major organizations providing MMT oversight	• roles and responsibilities of state methadone authority • roles and responsibilities of single state agency • use and roles of accrediting organizations
Licensure/certification procedures	• process application • types of certification required • demonstrate community needs assessment • community acceptance • prelicensure survey required • application to local authorities • evaluation criteria • resource requirements • length of license • grounds for revocation of license or certificate • appeals process
Monitoring/oversight	• inspections (oversight) • reporting requirements
Personnel	• staff training/education requirements • continued training/education requirements • staffing ratios • HIV/AIDS staff training
Patient record maintenance	• storage • treatment documentation • confidentiality
Medication requirements	• storage • record documentation • policies to prevent diversion • hours of operation
Treatment requirements	• services available • admissions • waiting list • medication units • maintenance (take-home policies) • detoxification • urinalysis testing • case review • patient rights
Service and evaluation processes	• prioritization • QA plans/procedures • program outcome/evaluation

- Use of accrediting organizations in licensing/regulating MMT programs

- Emphasis on QA plans and procedures

- Staffing ratio requirements

- Urinalysis testing

- Program/outcome evaluation

A detailed examination of these five dimensions found that all of the 14 states studied had at least one requirement that was different from the federal regulations. Four states addressed use of accrediting organizations in licensing/regulating MMT programs, seven emphasized QA plans and procedures, eight had staffing ratio requirements that went beyond the federal requirements, six had additional requirements for urinalysis testing, and six had additional regulations addressing program/outcome evaluation.

This analysis was based on a review of written state regulations and additional documents. The characterization of state regulatory approaches as more or less comprehensive was based only on the dimensions identified. Alternative characterizations might emerge, depending on whether other criteria are selected to characterize states. The dimensions identified were deemed important at a particular regulatory juncture (before the final accreditation rule), although many of the regulations reviewed had been in effect for some time.

In addition, this analysis does not address the application and implementation of the formal regulations by states, as some state administrative bodies may opt to adhere rigidly to the guidelines; others may have strong regulatory structures but may not administer them in their entirety. State regulations often lag behind actual policy, as in Michigan, which used an accreditation-based regulatory system, although this policy was not reflected in the state regulations.

To better understand variations in state regulation, it would be necessary to ascertain the extent to which state policies reflect state regulations. Many regulations are open to interpretation. For example, some requirements, such as QA plans and processes, may be interpreted with differing levels of rigor. Depending on a particular state's interpretation of the regulations, the impact on programs can be significant.

HOW DOES STATE FUNDING WORK WITH STATE REGULATION?

State funding of MMT is a powerful, nonregulatory method of creating and enforcing requirements for MMT programs. State funding includes both Medicaid funding and state funding through block grant monies. Various requirements generally accompany state funds; some examples follow.

In Indiana, the two state-funded programs were financed through a managed care arrangement, with a separate application for MMT. Providers were required to submit periodic reports and assessments, and only nonprofit MMT programs were eligible for state funding. State contracts included requirements for staffing and continuum of care that went beyond the federal requirements.

In Massachusetts, Medicaid funded MMT through a behavioral health carve-out. It increased the credentialing requirement for staff, which was linked to a higher reimbursement rate. Medicaid contracts included performance specifications, paperwork requirements, and authorization requirements; these may exceed the licensing requirements.

Nevada's state-funded programs were subject to annual program compliance monitoring visits. They were required to provide services on a state-approved sliding fee scale and follow mandatory reporting requirements, including a patient data system, fiscal reporting, and auditing.

In New York, 80% of the programs received funding from the state substance abuse office. Proprietary programs were not eligible for state monies but may have received Medicaid payments (although at a different reimbursement rate). Requirements of state-funded programs included annual cost and visit reports and admission and discharge reports, in accordance with the state registry standards.

WHAT DO STATES THINK ABOUT REGULATORY CHANGE?

In a prospective study of five states' anticipated reactions to a federal accreditation regulatory model, most respondents were generally positive about the shift to an accreditation-based system but had concerns about some aspects of the change. Few viewed the process as strictly positive or strictly negative, and those who did either lacked knowledge about accreditation or based their opinions on misinformation. For example, one respondent believed that office-based MMT would replace the clinic system. Another feared that counselors would lose their jobs to doctors and nurses under the new regulatory system.

Several state respondents were hopeful that accreditation would help normalize MMT. This normalization would benefit patients by bringing methadone into the mainstream treatment community, and it would enable providers to develop partnerships with other substance abuse and mental health programs so that patients could receive all necessary care.

Respondents were also enthusiastic about the conceptual changes that an accreditation model would offer, given its focus on quality and best practices at the clinic level. They believed this would support treatment decisions based on sound clinical judgment as opposed to law and regulations.

The new take-home regulations were seen as benefiting patients by allowing more flexibility and freedom. Greater use of take-home medications would also allow MMT programs to focus their resources on patients who were not stabilized and may need more clinical time.

Cost was one of the greatest concerns. Because most MMT providers have limited resources, some respondents feared that accreditation costs might be passed on to patients through rate increases. Others voiced concern that the cost to patients would be in clinical time if counselors were required to perform more administrative tasks, such as paperwork and training staff.

One of the most problematic issues was that states and providers did not know for certain how much accreditation would cost. Many gave examples of figures they had been given that heightened their concern.

Another common concern was the accreditation standards. Some respondents questioned whether an accrediting body such as JCAHO, which mainly accredits hospitals and inpatient facilities, had the knowledge and experience to develop and implement practical standards for MMT clinics.

HOW DO LOCAL JURISDICTIONS REGULATE MMT?

In some states, state regulations necessitate coordination with local entities. In New York, for example, MMT programs are required to contact the local government unit (usually the county) with regard to needs assessment and how the program fits into the county's chemical dependence plan. In Massachusetts, state legislation mandates a siting analysis, wherein applicant programs are required to provide notification of their intent to operate an MMT program to legislators, police, elected officials, community leaders, and owners of abutting properties. Pennsylvania has a zoning statute that prescribes the procedures a municipality must follow before it can grant zoning approval to an MMT facility within 500 feet of an existing school, public playground, public park, residential housing area, child care facility, or place of religious worship.

Local jurisdictions may also institute separate requirements for MMT programs; zoning requirements, in particular, can have a significant impact on program operations (CSAT, 2005).

SUMMARY

- MMT programs are subject to a wide range of regulatory oversight.

- State and local regulatory structures and processes are often complex and subject to change.

- The main challenge for MMT programs is to monitor and respond to regulatory oversight from entities that may not be fully coordinated with one another.

CHAPTER 12—Summary and Future Challenges

The Evaluation Study was conducted at a critical juncture in the history of MMT, when federal oversight was shifting from a traditional regulatory model based on compliance to an accreditation model based on maximizing quality of care. The findings from this study have provided important insights into the evolution of MMT, many of which we have tried to capture in this handbook. The study showed, for example, that many aspects of MMT have remained stagnant and that the negative perception of MMT has remained widespread in spite of the evidence documenting the treatment's effectiveness. This chapter highlights both the promising developments and the areas of lingering concern in the MMT field.

WHAT IS THE CURRENT STATE OF MMT?

In preparing this book, we focused on specific aspects of MMT within various types of programs. Although it is beneficial and informative to examine these individual aspects of MMT, it is essential to also examine the state of the field as a whole.

The growth of the MMT field reflects both the ongoing problem of opiate dependence and the increased demand for effective treatment. MMT has evolved on multiple dimensions over the past 40 years, and it has demonstrated its market value, as for-profit organizations are now opening clinics at a faster pace than nonprofit programs. States have also started contracting with for-profit programs to provide services. Nonprofit/public stand-alone programs are quickly becoming the minority; some have closed, and others have survived by becoming part of larger organizational entities. Multiple programs are now managed by a parent organization within and across states.

The Evaluation Study findings show that many programs are dedicated to their patients' recovery, providing a full array of support services in addition to pharmacologic treatment. The findings also show, however, that MMT programs vary considerably in how they assess patients, both at intake and through monitoring of patient functioning and outcomes.

Not all MMT programs have embraced the medical maintenance treatment model. Some programs continue to place an administrative upper limit on dosing, and the average dosage remains well below the recommended therapeutic dosage of 60 to 120 mg a day. In addition, limited availability of take-home doses constrains many MMT patients and keeps them from engaging fully in normal lives.

Overall, the Evaluation Study findings suggest that although MMT may be growing as an industry, there is still a critical need to ensure that programs provide patients with a standard quality of care grounded in a medical model of treatment. To that end, the MMT field should look forward to the changing regulatory oversight system and the implementation of accreditation to focus on improving standards of care.

IS MMT BECOMING A STREAMLINED SERVICE?

One model of MMT is to provide a broad array of patient services, including specialized care for subpopulations (e.g., pregnant women) and for patients with co-occurring conditions, as well as child care and transportation to clinics. However, this level of care may be becoming less common, in part because of the rapid expansion of MMT concurrent with the upsurge of HIV/AIDS in the 1980s and 1990s. The influx of HIV-positive patients into MMT programs in the 1980s at first meant that MMT programs were the frontline of medical service delivery. But as the number of MMT patients increased, programs often struggled to keep pace with the demand for additional services. The result was a streamlined system dependent on referral agencies to deliver a variety of ancillary services.

Although many services are available to MMT patients, they are often available only off-site and through links to other programs and service providers. One-stop, comprehensive services that would likely minimize patients' chances of failing to get the services they need may not be economically feasible under current funding structures and given patient demands. Committed service providers face these challenges as they try to ensure patient access to needed services.

Another factor influencing MMT service delivery is the varying needs of patients. These needs are no longer homeostatic but rather span a continuum, and comprehensive treatment programs may no longer be relevant for all patients. Streamlined models of MMT, which focus on pharmacologic treatment alone, are part of the new era of MMT, as is treatment in office-based practices. Policy makers need to monitor these developments to ensure that patients with multifaceted needs will continue to have services available to them, while not administratively overburdening programs that serve patients who need only pharmacologic treatment.

HOW WILL FDA APPROVAL OF BUPRENORPHINE CHANGE THE LANDSCAPE OF OPIATE DEPENDENCE TREATMENT?

In addition to the rising number of heroin initiates each year, the number of pain medication abusers is rising. According to national household data, the number of survey respondents reporting first-time nonmedical use of pain medications rose from 600,000 in 1990 to over 2 million in 2002. Possibly more alarming, however, is the continued rise of opiate use among youth and young adults. The 2004 NSDUH estimate of 4.4 million current nonprescription opiate users tells only part of the story. According to NSDUH estimates, in 2002, almost 30 million Americans aged 12 or older (13%) had used prescription pain relievers nonmedically at least once in their lifetime.

Current federal and state regulations allow MMT programs to treat only patients who have a diagnosis of opiate dependence and a history of at least 1 year of opiate abuse. This restriction discourages many individuals from seeking treatment, particularly those who have only recently become dependent on opiates. These recently dependent individuals are often the very individuals who could benefit the most from early intervention, especially in the face of increased opiate use among youth and young adults.

The regulations restricting access to MMT have resulted in a treatment system predominated by large urban MMT programs that provide care to long-term opiate-dependent patients through daily doses. MMT programs in the United States can provide for about 200,000 patients total and reach approximately 14% of opiate-dependent patients. The increasing number of persons using and abusing opiates, coupled with the limited availability of

MMT, demonstrates the need to expand both the access to and variety of treatments currently available to opiate addicts.

Buprenorphine treatment, offered in an office-based practice setting, provides patients with several advantages. Treatment in office-based practices has the potential to reach at least some of the nearly 85% of opiate-dependent patients who remain untreated each year, including newly dependent youth and young adults and residents of small rural communities who would otherwise be unable to access treatment. The use of buprenorphine in office-based practices aims to increase access to treatment for the hundreds of thousands of opiate-dependent patients who go untreated each year. Treatment in an office-based practice setting also serves to move opiate treatment into mainstream medicine, both legitimizing it and providing opiate-dependent patients with physicians able to address the conditions that often accompany opiate addiction (e.g., hepatitis C, HIV, depression). Finally, receiving care from physicians in an office-based setting removes much of the stigma associated with opiate treatment and decreases patients' contact with other addicts, which can increase the risk of relapse.

Buprenorphine offered through MMT programs also provides patients with beneficial alternatives to traditional methadone dosing. For example, buprenorphine can be used in less-than-daily dosing regimens because of its long duration of action, and its low abuse potential makes it more appealing for 30-day take-home prescriptions. To offer buprenorphine, MMT programs are required to review their state licensing laws and regulations and modify their registration with DEA to add Schedule III narcotics to their registration certificates.

Despite evidence of buprenorphine's efficacy and its benefit of increasing access to MMT, reports indicate that it is not in widespread use for the treatment of opiate addiction in either office-based practices or MMT programs. Nearly 35% of eligible physicians reported not prescribing buprenorphine at all, and other physicians reported several barriers to its use (e.g., availability of medication through pharmacies, high cost of medication, lack of practice protocols). Over 1,000 physicians serving as medical directors in MMT programs across the United States are eligible to use buprenorphine in the treatment of opiate addiction. The majority of physicians, however, have not yet applied to DEA on behalf of their treatment program to request eligibility, and no data are available on whether they are prescribing buprenorphine to their patients.

Although receiving FDA approval of buprenorphine treatment after years of delays marks a major advance, experiences with other FDA-approved pharmaceutical medications for use in opiate treatment (e.g., LAAM) have shown that this approval does not ensure utilization of buprenorphine. If buprenorphine is to meet its potential to increase access to opiate treatment, we need to understand the barriers to its adoption as a treatment modality.

HOW CAN MMT CONTINUE TO PLAY A ROLE IN REDUCING THE SPREAD OF HIV AND HCV?

MMT provides a good opportunity to address illnesses comorbid with opiate dependence, including HIV and HCV. Available treatment may vary by region; but, in general, new treatment for HCV is progressing rapidly, and ARV is available for most patients thanks to AIDS clinical trials with new regimens as well as Ryan White funding. For people living with HIV in the United States, access to treatment has become much less of a problem than it was several years ago. Despite the positive outlook on the availability of treatment for HIV and HCV, however, it is important to note that access to treatment remains variable and that treatment philosophy is inconsistent. As discussed earlier, MMT does not consistently offer direct access to ancillary medical services and often requires patients to transfer to a referral organization to receive necessary services.

Additionally, despite evidence that a harm-reduction approach can help control risk behaviors associated with drug use, including risks of both HIV and HCV, opposition persists toward any treatment model that does not view abstinence as the ultimate goal. The Evaluation Study findings suggest that treatment philosophies and approaches differ across MMT programs. The concept of harm reduction is misunderstood and highly political, often for the wrong reasons. Any strategy that offers alternatives for changing behavior in the right direction can be considered harm reduction. Regardless of how MMT is classified, the delivery of MMT services to help stabilize individuals in support of productive lives or reduction of risk behaviors continues to be an important aspect of public health care.

HOW WILL THE CHARACTERISTICS OF THE MMT PATIENT POPULATION CHANGE?

The traditional MMT patient population is aging; consequently, co-occurring physical health concerns will need to be addressed. The Evaluation Study findings suggest that many MMT programs will need to increase the availability of medical services and other supplementary services (e.g., transportation) to optimize patient health or ensure that links to services can provide guaranteed access. But newer evidence is also showing recent trends with youth abuse of prescription drugs. As a result of the increasing number of youth initiates of opiate abuse, the median patient age may decrease, and treatment service delivery may need to be adapted to reach a younger generation.

WHAT DOES THE FUTURE HOLD FOR MMT PROFESSIONALS?

With the exception of physicians, most social service professionals are women, perhaps because of salary limitations and because women may be drawn to service-oriented professions.

The Evaluation Study findings show that minority staff tend to have lower-paying positions (e.g., intake workers, administrative assistants). Clinical and medical director staff positions were generally filled by staff with the highest level of education. Nurses reported the lowest level of education; most had completed the requirements for an associate's degree or a certification as an LPN. The limited education among frontline nursing staff is somewhat troubling given nurses' integral role in daily dosing. Nurses were also found to have the most limited access to training opportunities.

Staff retention in many MMT programs is a major problem. This may be a function of low pay and poor benefits, which are typical in social service occupations, as well as a lack of opportunities for professional development. Nurses, counselors, and other staff play a critical role in caring for MMT patients. A greater investment in these staff members' professional growth and development on the part of MMT programs could improve staff retention and, in so doing, increase the likelihood of developing and sustaining good therapeutic relationships.

Several other Evaluation Study findings raised concerns about future staffing of MMT programs. First, staff are aging; more than half were 45 or older. In addition, only half were credentialed in substance abuse treatment, and many had limited experience in MMT. The implementation of accreditation standards requiring documentation of staff certification and training may either force a segment of professional staff out of the field or lead to significant retraining efforts. If it does reinforce the professional nature of the work, however, accreditation may help attract new staff to the MMT field.

Investing in appropriate salaries, benefits, staff development and training, and other ways of rewarding staff will be necessary for the field to achieve increased professionalism. But there is a cost for all of this, and the question is who will pay? Ultimately, MMT program administrators and advocates will need to work with state and federal governments to ensure appropriate reimbursement for the services they provide.

WILL THE QUALITY OF CARE CHANGE?

Accreditation of MMT programs is intended to increase the quality of care by reinforcing high standards. The Evaluation Study findings show that nearly all MMT programs had some QA measures in place, although many of these measures were in the early stages of development.

In the substance abuse treatment field, performance measurement is increasingly important for accountability and quality improvement. Although the field is far from adopting the pay-for-performance approach that is becoming increasingly common in general medical care, substance abuse treatment providers are aware of the need to be accountable to funders. The federal government is engaging in a national performance measurement effort—the State Outcomes Measurement and Management System—and MMT providers would do well to be active participants in this process to ensure that resulting outcomes are applicable to MMT.

WHAT IMPACT DOES STIGMATIZATION HAVE ON THE FUTURE OF MMT?

Throughout its four decades of existence and despite its demonstrated value and effectiveness, MMT has struggled to mitigate the stigma associated with opiate dependence and this treatment modality. It is well established that MMT can help stabilize patients, decrease criminal activity, and increase employment, yet public misperceptions of MMT programs persist (e.g., that they are a hotbed of drug dealing). Additionally, there is a persistent view of methadone as a harmful drug that is even harder to withdraw from than heroin. These views are often supported by misleading media coverage portraying MMT as a drug replacement rather than a rehabilitative therapy.

The notion that MMT trades dependence on heroin for dependence on methadone demonstrates a lack of understanding. Dependence is associated with continuing to engage in addictive behavior; MMT replaces this dependence with a pharmacologic alternative. Because methadone does not produce euphoria, the compulsive overuse that is a hallmark of heroin addiction is rarely a problem. The continuing controversy suggests a need for more effective public education campaigns to normalize MMT and overcome the stigma associated with it.

This, in turn, would help facilitate the opening of new MMT programs, which nearby neighborhoods often resist. When MMT programs are relegated to neighborhoods with less community mobilization, more social service providers, and more criminal activity, it becomes difficult to determine the causal links: is there more crime in a blighted neighborhood because an MMT program is there, or is the MMT program there because the blighted neighborhood is unlikely to organize opposition to it?

Additionally, in the large Evaluation Study sample of MMT clinics, the findings documented very little methadone diversion. Indeed, most instances of diversion are not attributable to patients. It is patients, however, who are stigmatized as a result of diversion. More effective attention to the security of methadone could do much to overcome this misconception.

HOW CAN LESSONS FROM OPIATE DEPENDENCE TREATMENT BE SHARED INTERNATIONALLY?

The international availability of MMT is increasing: treatment is now offered in the Netherlands, Switzerland, and the United Kingdom. Additionally, Australia, Canada, Denmark, Germany, and Spain are either considering offering MMT or are in initial implementation phases. These countries can benefit from the 40 years of experience in the United States. The complex, multitiered U.S. regulatory climate proved to be a treatment barrier for many years. Policy makers in other countries may find it expedient to adopt a more streamlined oversight policy, which may encourage greater treatment availability. Approaching MMT as a medical treatment for a chronic illness—with appropriate oversight, staffing, and reimbursement—will help normalize this effective treatment and alleviate the stigma that has historically shadowed MMT in the United States.

In addition to the increase of MMT availability, access to buprenorphine treatment for opiate dependence is also increasing. Currently, Australia, Austria, Belgium, the Czech Republic, Denmark, Finland, France, Great Britain, Germany, Greece, Hong Kong, Iceland, Italy, Luxembourg, Malaysia, Norway, Portugal, Singapore, the Slovak Republic, Sweden, and Switzerland all offer buprenorphine as a treatment modality. FDA recently approved buprenorphine treatment in the United States, and lessons from countries with established protocols and procedures for care may greatly enhance its utilization as an alternative to MMT.

Given the persistence of opiate dependence across cultures, open sharing of research and policy findings and implications could improve treatment and patient outcomes. The field of MMT should have an international focus, supporting a global initiative to address the ongoing problem of opiate addiction.

WHAT DOES THE FUTURE HOLD FOR MMT?

Opiate dependence is a worldwide problem, and the effectiveness of MMT has been clearly demonstrated. The data and findings presented here will serve to extend the MMT knowledge base and inform MMT programs, both in the United States and abroad, as the use of MMT continues to increase internationally.

To that end, the future of MMT holds a number of challenges, including

- ensuring that MMT offers access to a comprehensive array of support services for patients with co-occurring disorders

- investing in MMT program staff, mentoring them, and fostering their professional development to retain them in the field

- building collaborative relationships with local program administrators and federal legislators to reduce the current levels of oversight and bureaucracy for MMT services

- establishing an active and compelling voice within local communities, medical professions, and legislative bodies to counteract the persistent stigma associated with MMT.

A large and growing advocacy association of methadone professionals, the American Association for the Treatment of Opioid Dependence (AATOD), is committed to helping overcome these and other challenges. At this association's large annual conference, exhibitors, government speakers, and international participants learn about MMT best practices in the United States. In addition, MMT programs are now a business component of many hospitals and an aspect of office-based practices.

Glossary

abuse	According to the U.S. Food and Drug Administration, "deliberately taking a substance for other than its intended purpose, and in a manner that can result in damage to the person's health or his ability to function."
addiction	A behavioral syndrome characterized by the repeated, compulsive seeking or use of a substance despite adverse social, psychological, or physical consequences, and a need for an increased amount of the substance over time to achieve the same effect. Addiction is often accompanied by physical dependence, withdrawal syndrome, and tolerance.
administration	The means by which a drug is taken.
AIDS	Acquired immunodeficiency syndrome.
assessment	Systematic procedures for the identification of a client's major strengths and problem areas, culminating in a treatment plan and referral for assistance.
ceiling effect	The limiting of euphoria beyond a certain dosage.
client satisfaction	Formal survey of clients on satisfaction with various aspects of service.
detoxification	Metabolic process by which the body reduces the toxic qualities of a poison or toxin. Pertaining to addiction, it is generally a medically supervised treatment for alcohol or drug dependence, designed to purge the body of intoxicating or addictive substances. Such a program is used as a first step in overcoming physiological or psychological addiction.
Drug Addiction Treatment Act of 2000	Title XXXV of the Children's Health Act of 2000. The Drug Addiction Treatment Act of 2000 (DATA 2000) established a waiver authority for qualifying physicians to prescribe or dispense specially approved Schedule III, IV, and V narcotic medications for the treatment of opiate dependence in clinical settings other than methadone maintenance treatment programs.
full opioid agonists	Agonists that stimulate activity at opiate receptors in the brain that are normally stimulated by naturally occurring opiates. Examples include morphine, methadone, oxycodone, hydrocodone, heroin, codeine, meperidine, propoxyphene, and fentanyl.

group counseling	Provision of treatment in a group format. May include group psychotherapy, as well as other types of groups, such as support groups and counseling groups.
guidelines	Orientation or expert advice regarding work, taking into account the legal and historical contexts of the work setting. Guidelines should evolve naturally over time and represent a partial balance between scientific knowledge and context without providing exhaustive information.
half-life	Amount of time required for half of the amount of a drug in the body to be removed.
harm reduction	Social policy that gives priority to diminishing the negative effects caused by drug use. Its roots are in a scientific public health protection model based on a humanitarian culture. Envisages intermediate objectives as an alternative to the final aim of complete abstinence. These objectives include limiting the harm produced even before users decide or attempt to stop using drugs.
hepatitis	Inflammation of the liver.
heroin	Morphine diluted with acetyls (diacetylmorphine).
maintenance	Stabilization period. A drug user stays on a maintenance medication dose indefinitely to prevent relapse and to suppress lingering cravings.
methadone	Synthetic opiate with action similar to that of morphine and heroin, except that withdrawal is more prolonged and less severe. Used in methadone maintenance treatment programs as a substitute for heroin in the treatment of addiction.
methadone maintenance treatment	Type of treatment for individuals who are addicted to heroin or other opiates (such as Percodan or OxyContin). Methadone is a safe and effective medication that acts as a stabilizer so that heroin users can return to daily life. It does not create a high and does not replace one drug addiction with another; methadone's effects are different from those of other opiates. Most people receive methadone daily from a clinic, where counseling and group meetings are also available.
mu opioid receptor	Receptor on the surface membrane of nerve cells that mediates opioid analgesia, tolerance, and addiction through drug-induced activation. When an opioid agonist, or partial agonist (e.g., buprenorphine), binds to a mu opioid receptor, a series of other proteins associated with the mu receptor signals the pathway is activated. Other opioid receptors are the delta and kappa receptors.
needle exchange program	Free exchange of used or clean needles and other materials required for the safer injection of drugs (e.g., bleach kits).

opiate/opioid	Drug classified as a narcotic, either naturally or synthetically derived from opium (created from the seeds of the oriental poppy). Moderate to severe pain relievers are generally in this class of medication. Drug derived naturally from the flower of the opium poppy plant (e.g., morphine and heroin) or synthetically produced in a laboratory (e.g., methadone and oxycodone). Used therapeutically to treat pain but can produce euphoria—the narcotic high. Repeated misuse of opiates often leads to dependence and addiction.
opiate dependence	Subset of substance dependence (according to DSM-IV criteria) synonymous with and often used in place of "opioid addiction." A chronic brain disease that involves a physical, psychological, and behavioral need for an opioid drug. This need is unrelated to medical necessity for pain relief.
opioid agonist	Any opioid that produces morphine- or codeine-like effects on the body.
opioid antagonist	A drug that blocks the effects of an opiate. Used in cases of overdose and to show that a user is an addict, usually for the purpose of admission into a methadone maintenance treatment program.
outcome evaluation	Investigation of the impact of services for clients (e.g., percentage of clients who reduce alcohol use by 80% for 12 months following treatment).
partial opioid agonists	Can both activate and block opiate receptors. Depending on the conditions, can produce effects similar to those of either agonists or antagonists. Buprenorphine is a partial opioid agonist.
polysubstance abuse	Concurrent use or abuse of multiple substances (e.g., drinking alcohol as well as smoking tobacco, snorting cocaine, inhaling glue fumes).
quality assurance	Systematic process designed to maintain satisfactory levels of service delivery and to improve quality of care.
relapse	Resumption of drug-seeking or drug-taking behavior after a period of abstinence. Priming, environmental cues (people, places, or things associated with past drug use), and stress can trigger intense craving and cause a relapse.

take-home dose	Daily dose of methadone prescribed for a patient and approved for administration at home (rather than at an MMT clinic). Take-home doses provide stable patients with more flexibility by removing the need to present at the methadone maintenance treatment clinic daily for their medication. Take-home doses, however, are approved only for patients meeting certain criteria and for no more then 30 days at a time.
tolerance	The body's diminishing responsiveness to a substance with repeated use, requiring greater doses of a drug to achieve the same effect.
withdrawal	Predictable group of signs and symptoms resulting from abrupt removal of, or rapid decrease in, the regular dosage of a psychoactive substance. Often characterized by overactivity of the physiological functions that were suppressed by the substance or depression of the functions that were stimulated by the substance.

Appendix A: Opiates and Opioids

Generic Drug Name	Trade Name	Description
Opiates		
Opium	Pantopon, Laudanum	Extracted from the unripe seeds of the opium poppy (*Papaver somniferum*) of Southwestern Asia, an addictive narcotic that contains several alkaloids, including morphine (one of the most powerful natural painkillers and addictive narcotics known) and codeine (a milder painkiller). A more potent derivative of morphine. Sometimes given as a tincture dissolved in alcohol, known as laudanum. Opium also contains the highly poisonous alkaloid thebaine.
		There were no legal restrictions on the importation or use of opium until the early 1900s. In the United States, the unrestricted availability of opium, the influx of opium-smoking immigrants from East Asia, and the invention of the hypodermic needle contributed to the more severe variety of compulsive drug abuse seen at the turn of the 20th century. In those days, medicines often contained opium without any warning label. Today, there are state, federal, and international laws governing the production and distribution of narcotic substances.
		Although opium is used in the form of paregoric to treat diarrhea, most opium imported into the United States is broken down into its alkaloid constituents. These alkaloids are divided into two distinct chemical classes: phenanthrenes and isoquinolines. The principal phenanthrenes are morphine, codeine, and thebaine. Isoquinolines have no significant central nervous system effects and are not regulated under the Controlled Substances Act (CSA).

Opiates and Opioids *(continued)*

Generic Drug Name	Trade Name	Description
Opiates		
Morphine	Infumorph, Kadian, Roxanol	Principal constituent of opium; can range in concentration from 4% to 21%. Commercial opium is standardized to contain 10% morphine. In the United States, a small percentage of the morphine obtained from opium is used directly (about 15 tons); the remaining opium is converted to codeine and other derivatives (about 120 tons).
		Morphine is one of the most effective drugs known for the relief of severe pain and remains the standard against which new analgesics are measured. As with most narcotics, the use of morphine has increased significantly in recent years. Since 1990, there has been about a threefold increase in morphine products in the United States.
		Morphine is marketed in generic and brand-name products. It is used parenterally (by injection) for preoperative sedation, as a supplement to anesthesia, and for analgesia. It is the drug of choice for relieving pain from myocardial infarction and for its cardiovascular effects in the treatment of acute pulmonary edema.
		Traditionally, morphine was used almost exclusively by injection. Today, morphine is marketed in a variety of forms, including oral solutions, immediate and sustained-release tablets and capsules, suppositories, and injectable preparations. The availability of high-concentration morphine preparations (e.g., 20-mg/ml oral solutions, 25-mg/ml injectable solutions, and 200-mg sustained-release tablets) partially reflects the use of this substance for chronic pain management in opiate-tolerant patients.

Opiates and Opioids *(continued)*

Generic Drug Name	Trade Name	Description
Opiates		
Codeine	Empirin with codeine, Tylenol with codeine, Doriden with codeine	The most widely prescribed naturally occurring narcotic in the world, this alkaloid is found in opium in concentrations ranging from 0.7% to 2.5%. Most codeine used in the United States is produced from morphine. It is the starting material for the production of two other narcotics, dihydrocodeine and hydrocodone.
		Codeine is prescribed for the relief of moderate pain and for cough suppression. Compared with morphine, codeine produces less analgesia, sedation, and respiratory depression, and it is usually taken orally. It is made into tablets either alone (Schedule II) or in combination with aspirin or acetaminophen (e.g., Tylenol with codeine, Schedule III). As a cough suppressant, codeine is found in a number of liquid preparations, which are in Schedule V. Also used to a lesser extent as an injectable solution for the treatment of pain. Codeine products are diverted from legitimate sources and are found on the illicit market.
Thebaine	None	Minor constituent of opium, controlled in Schedule II of the CSA as well as under international law. Although chemically similar to both morphine and codeine, it produces stimulatory rather than depressant effects. Not used therapeutically but is converted into a variety of substances, including oxycodone, oxymorphone, nalbuphine, naloxone, naltrexone, and buprenorphine. The United States ranks first in the world in thebaine use.

Opiates and Opioids *(continued)*

Generic Drug Name	Trade Name	Description
Semisynthetic Opiates		
Diacetylmorphine	heroin	Semisynthetic drug derived from morphine. Discovered in 1874, introduced commercially in 1898 by the Bayer company in Germany. The name "heroin" was coined from the German "heroisch," meaning "heroic, strong." Heroin is stronger (more potent) than morphine and is considered a hard drug; intravenous injection provides the fastest and most intense rush.
Hydrocodone	Vicodin, Hycodan, Lortab, Lorcet, Zydone, Norco	Opioid agonist Schedule II narcotic. Mild to moderate analgesic and antitussive. Orally active and marketed in multi-ingredient Schedule III products. Has an analgesic potency similar to or greater than that of oral morphine. Sales and production have increased significantly in recent years (fourfold between 1990 and 2000), as have diversion and illicit use. Generally, abused by oral rather than intravenous administration.
Hydromorphone	Dilaudid	Marketed in tablets (2, 4, and 8 mg), rectal suppositories, oral solutions, and injectable formulations. All products are in Schedule II of the CSA. Hydromorphone's analgesic potency is 2 to 8 times that of morphine, but it is shorter acting and produces more sedation than morphine. Much sought after by narcotic addicts, hydromorphone is usually obtained by abusers through fraudulent prescriptions or theft. The tablets are often dissolved and injected as a substitute for heroin.
Oxycodone	Percodan, Tylox, OxyContin	Narcotic analgesic used in the treatment of moderate to severe pain. Adverse reactions include drowsiness, dizziness, nausea, constipation, respiratory and circulatory depression, and addiction.

Opiates and Opioids *(continued)*

Generic Drug Name	Trade Name	Description
Synthetic Opiates (Opioids)		
Methadone	Dolophine	Methadone hydrochloride is a synthetic narcotic analgesic with multiple actions quantitatively similar to morphine. The principal actions of therapeutic value are analgesia and sedation, and detoxification or maintenance in narcotic addiction.
		German scientists synthesized methadone during World War II because of a shortage of morphine. Although chemically unlike morphine or heroin, methadone produces many of the same effects. Introduced into the United States in 1947 as an analgesic (Dolophine), it is primarily used today for the treatment of narcotic addiction. It is available in oral solutions, tablets, and injectable Schedule II formulations, and is almost as effective when administered orally as it is by injection.
		Methadone's effects can last up to 24 hours, thereby permitting once-a-day oral administration in heroin detoxification and maintenance programs. High-dose methadone can block the effects of heroin, thereby discouraging the continued use of heroin by addicts under treatment with methadone. Chronic administration of methadone results in the development of tolerance and dependence. The withdrawal syndrome develops more slowly and is less severe but more prolonged than that associated with heroin withdrawal.

Opiates and Opioids *(continued)*

Generic Drug Name	Trade Name	Description
Synthetic Opiates (Opioids)		
Propoxyphene	Darvon, Darvocet-N, Wygesic	Mild, centrally acting narcotic analgesic structurally related to methadone, prescribed to relieve mild to moderate pain.
		A close relative of methadone, dextropropoxyphene was first marketed in 1957 under the trade name Darvon. Oral analgesic potency is one-half to one-third that of codeine (65 mg equivalent to about 600 mg of aspirin). Dextropropoxyphene is prescribed for relief of mild to moderate pain. Bulk dextropropoxyphene is in Schedule II; preparations containing it are in Schedule IV. This narcotic is associated with a number of toxic side effects, including liver dysfunction and depression of the central nervous system. It is among the top 10 drugs reported by medical examiners in drug abuse deaths.
Meperidine	Demerol, Mepergan	A narcotic analgesic used to treat moderate to severe pain and as a preoperative medication to relieve pain and reduce anxiety. Adverse reactions include respiratory and circulatory depression, dizziness, nausea, and dependence.
		Introduced as an analgesic in the 1930s, meperidine produces effects similar to those of morphine (with shorter duration and reduced antitussive and antidiarrheal actions). Currently, it is used for preanesthesia and the relief of moderate to severe pain, particularly in obstetrics and postoperative situations. Meperidine is available in tablets, syrups, and injectable forms under generic and brand-name (e.g., Demerol, Mepergan) Schedule II preparations. Several analogues of meperidine have been produced clandestinely.

Opiates and Opioids *(continued)*

Generic Drug Name	Trade Name	Description
Synthetic Opiates (Opioids)		
Fentanyl	Sublimaze, Duragesic, Actiq	A potent narcotic analgesic most commonly used as an appendage to general anesthesia or as a preoperative and postoperative painkiller; also prescribed to manage pain in cancer patients. Adverse effects include respiratory depression, circulatory depression, hypotension, and dependence.
		First synthesized in Belgium in the late 1950s, fentanyl, which has an analgesic potency about 80 times that of morphine, was introduced into medical practice in the 1960s as an intravenous anesthetic under the trade name Sublimaze. Thereafter, two other fentanyl analogues were introduced: alfentanil (Alfenta), an ultra-short-acting (5 to 10 minutes) analgesic, and sufentanil (Sufenta), an exceptionally potent analgesic (5 to 10 times more potent than fentanyl) for use in heart surgery. Today, fentanyl is used extensively for anesthesia and analgesia. Duragesic, for example, is a fentanyl transdermal patch used in chronic pain management, and Actiq is a solid formulation of fentanyl citrate on a stick that dissolves slowly in the mouth for transmucosal absorption. Actiq is intended for opiate-tolerant individuals and is effective in treating breakthrough pain in cancer patients. Carfentanil (Wildnil) is an analogue of fentanyl with an analgesic potency 10,000 times that of morphine. It is used in veterinary practice to immobilize large animals.
		Illicit use of pharmaceutical fentanyl first appeared in the mid-1970s in the medical community and continues to be a problem in the United States. To date, more than 12 analogues of fentanyl have been produced clandestinely and identified in U.S. drug traffic. The biological effects of fentanyl are indistinguishable from those of heroin, with the exception that fentanyl may be hundreds of times more potent. Fentanyl is most commonly used by intravenous administration, but like heroin, it can also be smoked or snorted.

Opiates and Opioids *(continued)*

Generic Drug Name	Trade Name	Description
Synthetic Opiates (Opioids)		
Pentazocine	Talwin	Developed in an effort to find or create an effective analgesic with less dependence-producing consequences. Introduced as an analgesic in 1967, pentazocine was frequently encountered in the illicit drug trade, usually in combination with tripelennamine, and added to Schedule IV of the CSA in 1979. An attempt at reducing the abuse of this drug was made with the introduction of Talwin Nx. This product contains a quantity of antagonist (naloxone) sufficient to counteract the morphine-like effects of pentazocine if the tablets are dissolved and injected.
Levorphanol	Levo-Dromoran	Narcotic analgesic used to relieve moderate to severe pain; can be habit forming.
Levo-alpha-acetylmethadol	LAAM	Closely related to methadone, this synthetic compound has an even longer duration of action (from 48 to 72 hours) than methadone, permitting a reduction in frequency of use. In 1994, it was approved as a Schedule II treatment drug for narcotic addiction. Both methadone and LAAM have high abuse potential. Their acceptability as narcotic treatment drugs is predicated on their ability to substitute for heroin, their long duration of action, and their oral mode of administration. This medicine is not a cure for addiction. It is used as part of an overall program that may include counseling, attending support group meetings, and other treatment recommended by a physician.
Buprenorphine	Buprenex	Semisynthetic narcotic derived from thebaine; being investigated for the treatment of narcotic addiction. Like methadone and LAAM, buprenorphine is potent (30 to 50 times the analgesic potency of morphine), has a long duration of action, and does not need to be injected. The buprenorphine products under development are sublingual tablets. Unlike the other treatment drugs, buprenorphine produces far less respiratory depression and is thought to be safer in overdose. It is currently available in the United States as an injectable Schedule V narcotic analgesic for human and veterinary use.

Opiates and Opioids *(continued)*

Generic Drug Name	Trade Name	Description
Synthetic Opiates (Opioids)		
Oxymorphone	Numorphan	An opioid analgesic with actions and uses similar to those of morphine, apart from an absence of cough suppressant activity. Used in the treatment of moderate to severe pain, including pain in obstetrics. May also be used as an adjunct to anesthesia.
Butorphanol	Stadol	A drug abused more often now that it is available as a nasal spray. Abuse of this product led to the 1997 control of butorphanol in Schedule IV of the CSA. Although butorphanol can be made from thebaine, it is usually manufactured synthetically.
Opioid Antagonists		
Naloxone	Narcan	Opioid antagonist that blocks the effects of endogenous and exogenous opioids. Effective in treating heroin or opioid overdose. When a heroin overdose victim is injected with the drug, opioid effects are reversed in a matter of seconds. Often, naloxone administration needs to be repeated until the heroin is completely metabolized by the body.
Naltrexone	Revia	Used to prevent relapse and to help break the cycle of opiate addiction. Taking naltrexone daily blocks the effects of heroin and any other opiate. Also used in detoxification and abstinence programs to reduce craving for alcohol and cocaine. A timed-release version of naltrexone (Naltrel), which would need to be injected only once a month, is being developed. Naltrexone is legally approved to treat heroin addiction.

Source: Drug Enforcement Administration, 2005; Inaba & Cohen, 2003.

References

Aceijas, C., Stimson, G. V., Hickman, M., & Rhodes, T. (2004). Global overview of injecting drug use and HIV infection among injecting drug users on behalf of the UN Reference Group on HIV/AIDS Prevention and Care among IDU in Developing and Transitional Countries. *AIDS, 18*(17), 2295–2303.

Ameen, A., Sullivan, K., Malhotra, D., Ringel, D., & Harwood, R. (1999). *An analysis of state methadone regulations from fourteen states.* Rockville, MD: Center for Substance Abuse Treatment.

Ball, J. C., & Ross, A. (1991). *The effectiveness of methadone maintenance treatment: Patients, programs, services, and outcomes.* New York: Springer-Verlag.

Berkman, N.D. & Wechsberg, W.M. (in press). Access to Treatment-Related and Support Services in Methadone Treatment Programs. *Journal of Substance Abuse Treatment.*

Brooner, R. K., King, V. L., Kidorf, M., Schmidt, C. W. Jr., & Bigelow, G. E. (1997). Psychiatric and substance use comorbidity among treatment-seeking opioid abusers. *Archives of General Psychiatry, 54*(1), 71–80.

Brown, L. S., Ajuluchukwu, D. C., Gonzalez, V., & Chu, A. F. (1992). *Medical disorders of female intravenous drug abusers in methadone maintenance treatment programs.* NIDA Special Monograph. Rockville, MD: U.S. Department of Health and Human Services.

California Department of Alcohol and Drug Programs. (2004). California Drug and Alcohol Treatment Assessment (CALDATA), 1991–1993 [Computer file]. Conducted by the National Opinion Research Center at the University of Chicago and Lewin-VHI, Inc. ICPSR ed. Ann Arbor, MI: Inter-university Consortium for Political and Social Research [producer and distributor].

Calsyn, D. A., Saxon, A. J., Blaes, P., & Lee-Meyer, S. (1990). Staffing patterns of American methadone maintenance programs. *Journal of Substance Abuse Treatment, 7*(4), 255–259.

Caplehorn, J. R., & Bell, J. (1991). Methadone dosage and retention of patients in maintenance treatment. *Medical Journal of Australia, 154*(3), 195–199.

Caplehorn, J. R., McNeil, D. R., & Kleinbaum, D. G. (1993). Clinic policy and retention in methadone maintenance. *International Journal of the Addictions, 28*(1), 73–89.

Caplehorn, J. R. M., Lumley, T. S., & Irwig, L. (1998). Staff attitudes and retention of patients in methadone maintenance programs. *Drug and Alcohol Abuse, 52*(1), 57–61.

Center for Substance Abuse Treatment. (1999). *CSAT guidelines for the accreditation of opioid treatment programs.* Rockville, MD: U.S. Department of Health and Human Services.

Center for Substance Abuse Treatment. (2001). *CSAT guidelines for the accreditation of opioid treatment programs—Amended.* Rockville, MD: U.S. Department of Health and Human Services.

Center for Substance Abuse Treatment. (2005). *Medication-assisted treatment for opioid addiction in opioid treatment programs.* Treatment Improvement Protocol (TIP) Series 43. (DHHS publication no. [SMA] 05-4048). Rockville, MD: Substance Abuse and Mental Health Services Administration.

Chatham, L. R., Hiller, M. L., Rowan-Szal, G. A., Joe, G. W., & Simpson, D. D. (1999). Gender differences at admission and follow-up in a sample of methadone maintenance clients. *Substance Use & Misuse, 34*(8), 1137–1165.

Chou, C.-P., Hser, Y.-I., & Anglin, M. D. (1998). Interaction effects of client and treatment program characteristics on retention: An exploratory analysis using hierarchical linear models. *Substance Use & Misuse, 33*(11), 2281–2301.

Chriqui, J. F., Eidson, S. K., McBride, D. C., Scott, W., Capaccia, V., & Chaloupka, F. J. (2006). *Assessing state regulation of outpatient substance abuse treatment along a quality continuum.* Research Paper Series, No. 34. Champaign, IL: University of Illinois at Chicago Press.

Commission on the Accreditation of Rehabilitation Facilities (1998). *Opioid treatment program accreditation standards manual.* Tucson, AZ: Commission on the Accreditation of Rehabilitation Facilities.

Community Epidemiology Work Group. (2006, January). *Epidemiologic trends in drug abuse: Advance report.* Baltimore, MD: National Institute on Drug Abuse (NIDA), National Institutes of Health (NIH), Department of Health and Human Services.

Condelli, W. S., Dunteman, G. H., & Fairbank, J. A. (1993). Do methadone patients substitute other drugs for heroin? Predicting substance use at 1-year follow-up. *American Journal of Drug and Alcohol Abuse, 19*(4), 465–472.

Cooper, J. R. (1989). Methadone treatment and acquired immunodeficiency syndrome. *Journal of the American Medical Association, 262*(12), 1664–1668.

Cooper-Patrick, L., Gallo, J. J., Gonzales, J. J., Vu, H. T., Powe, N. R., Nelson, C., & Ford, D. E. (1999). Race, gender, and partnership in the patient-physician relationship. *The Journal of the American Medical Association, 282*, 583–589.

Craddock, S. G., Hubbard, R. L., Rachal, J. V., & Ginzburg, H. M. (1981). *Pretreatment profiles of men and women entering drug abuse treatment in 1979: A comparative analysis.* Research Triangle Park, NC: Research Triangle Institute.

Curtis, B., & Simpson, D. D. (1976). Demographic characteristics of groups classified by patterns of multiple drug abuse: A 1969–1971 sample. *The International Journal of the Addictions, 11*(1), 161–173.

Czechowicz, D., Hubbard, R. L., Phillips, C. D., Fountain, D. L., Cooper, J. R., Molinari, S. P., Luckey, J. W., & Graham, L. A. (1997). Methadone Treatment Quality Assurance System (MTQAS): A federal effort to assess the feasibility of using outcome indicators for methadone treatment. *Journal of Maintenance in the Addictions, 1*(1), 11–24.

D'Aunno, T., Folz-Murphy, N., & Lin, X. (1999). Changes in methadone treatment practices: Results from a panel study, 1988–1995. *American Journal of Drug and Alcohol Abuse, 25*(4), 681–699.

D'Aunno, T., & Pollack, H. A. (2002). Changes in methadone treatment practices: Results from a national panel study, 1988–2000. *Journal of the American Medical Association, 288*(7), 850–856.

D'Aunno, T., & Vaughn, T. E. (1992). Variations in methadone treatment practices. Results from a national study. *Journal of the American Medical Association, 267*(2), 253–258.

D'Aunno, T., & Vaughn, T. E. (1995). An organizational analysis of service patterns in outpatient drug abuse treatment units. *Journal of Substance Abuse Treatment, 7*(1), 27–42.

D'Aunno, T., Vaughn, T. E., & McElroy, P. (1999). An institutional analysis of HIV prevention efforts by the nation's outpatient substance abuse treatment units. *Journal of Health and Social Behavior, 40*(2), 175–192.

Dole, V. P. (1988). Implications of methadone maintenance for theories of narcotic addiction. *Journal of the American Medical Association, 260*(20), 3025–3029.

Dole, V. P., & Nyswander, M. E. (1965). A medical treatment for diacetylmorphine (heroin) addiction. *Journal of the American Medical Association, 193,* 80–84.

Drug Enforcement Administration. (2005). *Drugs of abuse.* Retrieved on June 7, 2006, from http://www.usdoj.gov/dea/pubs/abuse/index.htm#Contents.

Ducharme, L. J. , & Luckey, J. W. (2000). Implementation of the methadone treatment quality assurance system. Findings from the feasibility study. *Evaluation & the Health Professions, 23*(1), 72–90.

Farrell, M., Ward, J., Mattick, R., Hall, W., Stimson, G. V., Des Jarlais, D., Gossop, M., & Strang, J. (1994). Methadone maintenance treatment in opiate dependence: a review. *British Medical Journal, 309*(6960), 997–1001.

Forman, R. F., Bovasso, G., & Woody, G. (2001). Staff beliefs about addiction treatment. *Journal of Substance Abuse Treatment, 21*(1), 1–9.

Friedmann, P. D., D'Aunno, T. A., Jin, L., & Alexander, J. A. (2000). Medical and psychosocial services in drug abuse treatment: Do stronger linkages promote client utilization? *Health Services Research, 35*(2), 443–465.

Friedmann, P. D., Lemon, S. C., Stein, M. D., Etheridge, R. M., & D'Aunno, T. A. (2001). Linkage to medical services in the Drug Abuse Treatment Outcome Study. *Medical Care, 39*(3), 284–295.

General Accounting Office. (1990). *Drug abuse research on treatment may not address current needs.* (Report No. GAO/HRD-90-114). Washington, DC: General Accounting Office.

General Accounting Office. (1990). *Methadone maintenance: Some programs are not effective: Greater federal oversight needed.* (Report No. GAO/HRD-90-104). Washington, DC: General Accounting Office.

Gerstein, D. R., Datta, A. R., Ingels, J. S., Johnson, R. A., Rasinski, K. A., Schildhaus, S., Talley, K., Jordan, K., Phillips, D. B., Anderson, D. W., Condelli, W. G., & Collins, J. S. (1997). *The National Treatment Improvement Evaluation Study—Final Report.* Rockville, MD: Substance Abuse and Mental Health Services Administration, Center for Substance Abuse Treatment.

Gerstein, D. R., Johnson, R.A., Larison, C.L., Harwood, H.J., & Fountain, D. (1997). *Alcohol and other drug treatment for parents and welfare recipients: Outcomes, costs, and benefits.* Final report (HHS-100-95-0036). Washington, DC: U.S. Department of Health and Human Services, Office of the Assistant Secretary for Planning and Evaluation.

Gowing, L. R., Farrell, M., Bornemann, R., Sullivan, L. E., & Ali, R. L. (2006). Methadone treatment of injecting opioid users for prevention of HIV infection. *Journal of General Internal Medicine, 21*(2), 193–195.

Gray, B., & Stoddard, J. J. (1997). Patient-physician pairing: does racial and ethnic congruity influence selection of a regular physician? *Journal of Community Health, 22*(4), 247–259.

Grella, C. E., Annon, J. J., & Anglin, M. D. (1995). Ethnic differences in HIV risk behaviors, self-perceptions, and treatment outcomes among women in methadone maintenance treatment. *Journal of Psychoactive Drugs, 27*(4), 421–433.

Hagan, H., Thiede, H., & Des Jarlais, D. C. (2005). HIV/hepatitis C virus co-infection in drug users: risk behavior and prevention. *AIDS, 19*(suppl 3), S199–S207.

Harrison, L. D., Backenheimer, M., & Inciardi, J. A. (1995). Cannabis use in the United States: implications for policy. In P. Cohen & A. Sas (Eds.), *Cannabisbeleid in Duitsland, Frankrijk en de Verenigde Staten.* Amsterdam: Centrum voor Drugsonderzoek, Universiteit van Amsterdam.

Heimer, R., & Abdala, N. (2000). Viability of HIV-1 in syringes: implications for interventions among injection drug users. *AIDS Reader, 10*(7), 410–417.

Heimer, R., Clair, S., Grau, L., Bluthenthal, R., Marshall, P., & Singer, M. (2002). Hepatitis-associated knowledge is low and risks are high among HIV-aware injection users in three US cities. *Addiction, 97*, 1277–1287.

Holmberg, S. D. (1996). The estimated prevalence and incidence of HIV in 96 large US metropolitan areas. *American Journal of Public Health, 86*, 643–654.

Horgan, C. M., & Merrick, E. L. (2001). Financing of substance abuse treatment services. *Recent Developments in Alcoholism, 15*, 229–252.

Hser, Y.-I., Anglin, M. D., & Booth, M. W. (1987). Sex differences in addict careers. 3. Addiction. *American Journal of Drug and Alcohol Abuse, 13*(3), 231–251.

Hubbard, R. L., Marsden, M. E., Rachal, J. V., Harwood, H. J., Cavanaugh, R. R., & Ginzburg, H. M. (1989). *Drug abuse treatment: A national study of effectiveness.* Chapel Hill, NC: University of North Carolina Press.

Inaba, D., & Cohen, W. E. (2003). *Uppers, downers, all arounders* (5th ed.). Ashland, OR: CNS Publications.

Joe, G. W., Simpson, D. D., & Hubbard, R. L. (1991). Treatment predictors of tenure in methadone maintenance. *Journal of Substance Abuse, 3*(1), 73–84.

Joe, G. W., Simpson, D. D., & Sells, S. B. (1994). Treatment process and relapse to opioid use during methadone maintenance. *American Journal of Drug and Alcohol Abuse, 20*(2), 173–197.

Joe, G. W., Singh, B. K., Garland, J., Lehman, W., Sells, S. B., & Seder, P. (1983). Retention in outpatient drug free treatment clinics. *Addictive Behaviors, 8*(3), 219–234.

Joint Commission on Accreditation of Healthcare/Hospital Organizations. (2000). *Comprehensive accreditation manual for behavioral health care, 2000 supplement.* Oakbrook Terrace, IL: Author.

Kelley, M. S. (2001). Toward an understanding of responses to methadone maintenance treatment organizational style. *Research in Social Problems and Public Policy, 8*, 247–273.

Kidorf, M., King, V. L., & Brooner, R. K. (1999). Integrating psychosocial services with methadone treatment. In Strain, E. C., & Stitzer, M. L. (eds.), *Methadone treatment for opioid dependence* (pp 166–195). Baltimore, MD: Johns Hopkins University Press.

Kosten, T. R., Rounsaville, B. J., & Kleber, H. D. (1985). Ethnic and gender differences among opiate addicts. *The International Journal of the Addictions, 20*(8), 1143–1162.

Kreek, M. J. (2000). Methadone-related opioid agonist pharmacotherapy for heroin addiction: History, recent molecular and neurochemical research and future in mainstream medicine. *Annals of the New York Academy of Sciences, 909,* 186–216.

Latkin, C. A., Forman-Hoffman, V. L., D'Souza, G., & Knowlton, A. R. (2004). Associations between medical service use and HIV risk among HIV-positive drug users in Baltimore, MD. *AIDS Care, 16,* 901–908.

Leavitt, S. B., Shinderman, M., Maxwell, S., Eap, C. B., & Paris, P. (2000). When "enough" is not enough: New perspectives on optimal methadone maintenance dose. *Mt Sinai Journal of Medicine, 67*(5–6), 404–411.

Levine, H. J., Reif, S., Lee, M. T., Ritter, G. A., & Horgan, C. M. (2004). *The national treatment system: Outpatient methadone facilities.* Report of the Alcohol and Drug Services Study (ADSS). Office of Applied Studies, Substance Abuse and Mental Health Services Administration, Department of Health and Human Services.

Ling, W., Wesson, D. R., Charuvastra, C., & Klett, C. J. (1996). A controlled trial comparing buprenorphine and methadone maintenance in opioid dependence. *Archives of General Psychiatry,* 53(5), 401–407.

Magura, S., Nwakeze, P. C., Kang, S. Y., & Demsky, S. (1999). Program quality effects on patient outcomes during methadone maintenance: A study of 17 clinics. *Substance Use and Misuse, 34*(9), 1299–1324.

Mallinckrodt Inc. (1995). *Methadose® oral tablets* (Methadone hydrochloride tablets USP; 5, 10, 40 mg) [package inserts]. St. Louis, MO: Mallinckrodt Inc.

Mallinckrodt Inc. (2000). *Methadose® oral concentrate* (Methadone hydrochloride oral concentrate USP) [package insert]. St. Louis, MO: Mallinckrodt Inc.

Maremmani, I., Nardini, R., Zolesi, O., & Castrogiovanni, P. (1994). Methadone dosages and therapeutic compliance during a methadone maintenance program. *Drug and Alcohol Dependence, 34*(2), 163–166.

Mark, H. D., Nanda, J., Davis-Vogel, A., Navaline, H., Scotti, R., Wickrema, R., Metzger, D., & Sochalski, J. (2006). Profiles of self-reported HIV-risk behaviors among injection drug users in methadone maintenance treatment, detoxification, and needle exchange programs. *Public Health Nursing, 23*(1), 11–19.

Marsh, K. L., & Simpson, D. D. (1986). Sex differences in opioid addiction careers. *The American Journal of Drug and Alcohol Abuse, 12*(4), 309–329.

Mason, B. J., Kocsis, J. H., Melia, D., Khuri, E. T., Sweeney, J., Wells, A., Borg, L., Millman, R. B., & Kreek, M. J. (1998). Psychiatric comorbidity in methadone maintained patients. *Journal of Addictive Diseases, 17*(3), 75–89.

McCaughrin, W. C. (1991). Antecedents of optimal decision making for client care in health services delivery organizations. *Medical Care Review, 48*(3), 331–362.

McCaughrin, W. C., & Price, R. H. (1992). Effective outpatient drug treatment organizations: Program features and selection effects. *International Journal of the Addictions, 27*(11), 1335–1358.

McLellan, A. T., Arndt, I. O., Metzger, D. S., Woody, G. E., & O'Brien, C. P. (1993). The effects of psychosocial services in substance abuse treatment. *The Journal of the American Medical Association, 269*(15), 1953–1959.

McLellan, A. T., Kushner, H., Metzger, D., Peters, R., Smith, I., Grissom, G., Pettinati, H., & Argeriou, M. (1992). The Fifth Edition of the Addiction Severity Index. *Journal of Substance Abuse Treatment, 9*(3), 199–213.

Metzger, D. S., & Platt, J. J. (1987). Methadone dose levels and client characteristics in heroin addicts. *International Journal of the Addictions, 22*(2), 187–194.

Metzger, D. S., Woody, G. E., McLellan, A. T., O'Brien, C. P., Druley, P., Navaline, H., DePhilippis, D., Stolley, P., & Abrutyn, E. (1993). Human immunodeficiency virus seroconversion among intravenous drug users in- and out-of-treatment: An 18-month prospective follow-up. *Journal of Acquired Immune Deficiency, 6*(9), 1049–1056.

Narcotic Addiction Treatment Act. (1974). Pub. L. 93-281, 88 Stat. 124.

National Institute on Drug Abuse. (1999). *Principles of drug addiction treatment: A research-based guide.* Baltimore, MD: NIDA.

National Institutes of Health. (1997). Effective medical treatment of opiate addiction. *NIH Consensus Statement, 15*(6), 1–38.

Neaigus, A., Gyarmathy, A., Miller, M., Frajzyngier, V. M., Friedman, S. R., & Des Jarlais D. C. (2006). Transitions to injecting drug use among noninjecting heroin users: social network influence and individual susceptibility. *Journal of Acquired Immune Deficiency Syndrome, 41*(4), 493–503.

Nurco, D. N., Hanlon, T. E., & Kinlock, T. W. (March 1990). *Offenders, drugs, crime and treatment: Literature review.* Washington, DC: U.S. Department of Justice, Bureau of Justice Assistance.

Office of Applied Studies. (1998). *1998 Services Research Outcomes Study (SROS).* Rockville, MD: Department of Health and Human Services, Substance Abuse and Mental Health Services Administration.

Office of Applied Studies. (2003). *Results from the 2002 National Survey on Drug Use and Health: National findings.* (DHHS publication no. [SMA] 03-3836, NSDUH Series H-22). Rockville, MD: Substance Abuse and Mental Health Services Administration.

Office of Applied Studies. (2004). *Results from the 2003 National Survey on Drug Use and Health: National findings.* (DHHS publication no. [SMA] 04-3964, NSDUH Series H-25). Rockville, MD: Substance Abuse and Mental Health Services Administration.

Office of Applied Studies. (2005). *Results from the 2004 National Survey on Drug Use and Health: National findings.* (DHHS publication no. [SMA] 05-4062, NSDUH Series H-28). Rockville, MD: Substance Abuse and Mental Health Services Administration.

Palepu, A., Tyndall, M. W., Joy, R., Kerr, T., Wood, E., Press, N., Hogg, R. S., & Montaner, J. S. G. (in press). Antiretroviral adherence and HIV treatment outcomes among HIV/HCV co-infected injection drug users: The role of methadone maintenance therapy. *Drug and Alcohol Dependence.*

The Palm Beach County Substance Abuse Coalition. (2005, June 14). *Generation Rx: National experts address local forum on prescription drug abuse, parents and professionals learn signs of abuse and how to deter it.* Press release.

Parrino, M. (1993). *State methadone treatment guidelines. Treatment improvement protocol series (TIPS) 1.* (DHHS publication no. [SMA] 93-1991). Washington, DC: U.S. Government Printing Office.

The Partnership for a Drug-Free America. (2005, April 21). *Partnership Attitude Tracking Study: Teens, 2004.*

Payte, J. T. (1997). Methadone maintenance treatment: The first thirty years. *Journal of Psychoactive Drugs, 29*(2), 149–153.

Phillips, C. D., Hubbard, R. L., Dunteman, G., Fountain, D. L., Czechowicz, D., & Cooper, J. R. (1995). Measuring program performance in methadone treatment using in-treatment outcomes: An illustration. *Journal of Mental Health Administration, 22*(3), 214–225.

Pugatch, D., Anderson, B. J., O'Connell, J. V., Elson, L., & Stein, M. (2006). HIV and HCV testing for young drug users in Rhode Island. *Journal of Adolescent Health, 38*, 302–304.

Rettig, R. A., & Yarmolinsky, A. (1995). *Federal regulation of methadone treatment.* Prepared by the Committee on Federal Regulation of Methadone Treatment, Division of Biobehavioral Sciences and Mental Disorders, Institute of Medicine.

Rosenbaum, M. (1995). The demedicalization of methadone maintenance. *Journal of Psychoactive Drugs, 27*(2), 145–149.

Roussel, A. E., Layton, C. M., & Squire, C. M. (2002). *Opioid treatment program accreditation project: Special study on state issues.* Rockville, MD: Center for Substance Abuse Treatment.

Rowan-Szal, G. A., Chatham, L. R., Joe, G. W., & Simpson, D. D. (2000). Services provided during methadone treatment. A gender comparison. *Journal of Substance Abuse Treatment, 19*(1), 7–14.

Saha, S., Leemis, R. H., Holdsworth, M. T., Anderson, J. R., Raisch, D. W., Hermos, J. A., Gilson, S. B., Morrison, R. S., Wallenstein, S., Freeman, H. P., & Payne, R. (2000). We don't carry that. *New England Journal of Medicine, 343*, 442–445.

Schiff, M., El-Bassel, N., Engstrom, M., & Gilbert, L. (2002). Psychological distress and intimate physical and sexual abuse among women in methadone maintenance treatment programs. *Social Service Review, 76*(2), 302–320.

Schottenfeld, R. S., Pakes, J. R., Oliveto, A., Ziedonis, D., & Kosten, T. R. (1997). Buprenorphine vs. methadone maintenance treatment for concurrent opioid dependence and cocaine abuse. *Archives of General Psychiatry, 54*(8), 713–720.

Schroeder, J. R., Epstein, D.H., Umbricht, A., & Preston, K.L. (2006). Changes in HIV risk behaviors among patients receiving combined pharmacological and behavioral interventions for heroin and cocaine dependence. *Addictive Behaviors, 31*(5), 868-879.

Seivewright, N. (2000). *Community treatment of drug misuse: More than methadone.* Cambridge, MA: Cambridge University Press.

Sells, S. B., & Simpson, D. D. (1976). *The effectiveness of drug abuse treatment* (vol. 3). Cambridge, MA: Ballinger.

Selwyn, P. A., Budner, N. S., Wasserman, W. C., & Arno, P. S. (1993). Utilization of on-site primary care services by HIV-seropositive and seronegative drug users in a methadone maintenance program. *Public Health Reports, 108*(4), 492–500.

Strain, E. C., Bigelow, G. E., Liebson, I. A., & Stitzer, M. L. (1999). Moderate- vs. high-dose methadone in the treatment of opioid dependence: A randomized trial. *Journal of the American Medical Association, 281*(11), 1000–1005.

Strain, E. C., Stitzer, M. L., Liebson, I. A., & Bigelow, G. E. (1993). Dose-response effects of methadone in the treatment of opioid dependence. *Annals of Internal Medicine, 119*(1), 23–7.

Strathdee, S. A., & Patterson T. L. (2006). Behavioral interventions for HIV-positive and HCV-positive drug users. *AIDS and Behavior, 10*(2), 115–130.

Substance Abuse and Mental Health Services Administration. (1998). *The Services Research Outcomes Study (SROS).* Rockville, MD: U.S. Department of Health and Human Services, Substance Abuse and Mental Health Services Administration.

Substance Abuse and Mental Health Services Administration, Office of Applied Studies. (2006). *Treatment Episode Data Set (TEDS). Highlights—2004. National Admissions to Substance Abuse Treatment Services.* (DASIS Series: S-31, DHHS publication no. [SMA] 06-4140). Rockville, MD: Author.

Tennant, F. (2001). Hepatitis C, B, D, and A: Contrasting features and liver function abnormalities in heroin addicts. *Journal of Addictive Diseases, 20*(1), 9–17.

Umbricht-Schneiter, A., Ginn, D. H., Pabst, K. M., & Bigelow, G. E. (1994). Providing medical care to methadone clinic patients: Referral vs. on-site care. *American Journal of Public Health, 84*(2), 207–210.

Unger, J. B., Kipke, M. D., De Rosa, C. J., Hyde, J., Ritt-Olson, A., & Montgomery, S. (in press). Needle-sharing among young IV drug users and their social network members: The influence of the injection partners' characteristics on HIV risk behavior. *Addictive Behaviors.*

U.S. Census Bureau (2000). *Census 2000.* Available at www.census.gov/main/www/cen2000. html.

U.S. Department of Health and Human Services. (1999). Narcotic drugs in maintenance and detoxification treatment of narcotic dependence; Repeal of current regulations and proposal to adopt new regulations; Proposed Rule. *Federal Register, 64*(140), 39809–39857.

U.S. Department of Health and Human Services. (2001a). Opioid drugs in maintenance and detoxification treatment of opiate addiction: Final rule. *Federal Register, 66*(11), 4076–4102.

U.S. Department of Health and Human Services. (2001b). *Year-End 2000 Emergency Department Data from the Drug Abuse Warning Network.* Rockville, MD: Office of Applied Studies, Substance Abuse and Mental Health Services Administration, U.S. Department of Health and Human Services.

U.S. Department of Health and Human Services, Substance Abuse and Mental Health Treatment Services Administration. (1997). *The National Treatment Improvement Evaluation Study (NTIES): Final report.* Rockville, MD: Office of Applied Studies, Substance Abuse and Mental Health Services Administration, U.S. Department of Health and Human Services, Center for Substance Abuse Treatment.

U.S. Food and Drug Administration. (1972). 21 CFR, part 291.501.

Vlahov, D., & Celentano, D. D. (2006). Access to highly active antiretroviral therapy for injection drug users: Adherence, resistance, and death. *Cadernos de Saúde Pública, 22*(4), 705–731.

Ward, J., Mattick, R. P., & Hall, W. (Eds.) (1998). *Methadone maintenance treatment and other opioid replacement therapies* (pp. 205–238). Amsterdam: Overseas Publishers Association, Harwood Academic Publishers.

Wechsberg, W. M., Cavanaugh, E. R., Dunteman, G. H., & Smith, F. J. (1994). Changing needle practices in community outreach and methadone treatment. *Evaluation and Program Planning, 17,* 371–379.

Wechsberg, W. M., Craddock, S. G., & Hubbard, R. L. (1998). How are women who enter substance abuse treatment different than men? A gender comparison from the Drug Abuse Treatment Outcome Study. *Drugs and Society, 13*(1&2), 97–115.

Wechsberg, W. M., Dennis, M., Cavanaugh, E., & Rachal, V. (1993). A comparison of injecting drug users reached through outreach and methadone treatment. *Journal of Drug Issues, 23*(4), 667–687.

Wechsberg, W. M., Flannery, B., Suerken, C., Dunlap, L., Roussel, A. E., Crum, L., Murdoch, O., & Diesenhaus, H. (2004). Physicians practicing in methadone programs: Who are they and what do they do? *Journal of Addictive Diseases, 23*(2), 15–31.

Wechsberg, W. M., Kasten, J. J., Bobashev, G., Zarkin, G., Berkman, N., Roussel, A., Dunlap, L., Crum, L., Flannery, B., & Fulmer, E. (August 2003). *The Opioid Accreditation Evaluation Study: Results and implications.* Final report. Rockville, MD: Center for Substance Abuse Treatment.

Wheeler, J. R., Fadel, H., & D'Aunno, T. A. (1992). Ownership and performance of outpatient substance abuse treatment centers. *American Journal of Public Health, 82*(5), 711–718.

Wheeler, J. R., & Nahra, T. A. (2000). Private and public ownership in outpatient substance abuse treatment: do we have a two-tiered system? *Administration and Policy in Mental Health, 27*(4), 197–209.

Wilkerson, D., Migas, N., & Slaven, T. (2000). Outcome-oriented standards and performance indicators for substance dependency rehabilitation programs. *Substance Use and Misuse, 35*(12–14), 1679–1703.

Zaric, G. S., Barnett, P. G., & Brandeau, M. L. (2000). HIV transmission and the cost-effectiveness of methadone maintenance. *American Journal of Public Health, 90*(7), 1–7.

Zarkin, G. A., Dunlap, L. J., Bray, J. W., & Wechsberg, W. M. (2002). The effect of treatment completion and length of stay on employment and crime in outpatient drug-free treatment. *Journal of Substance Abuse Treatment, 23*, 261–271.

Zarkin, G. A., Dunlap, L. J., & Homsi, G. (2004). The substance abuse services cost analysis program (SASCAP): A new method for estimating drug treatment services costs. *Evaluation and Program Planning, 2*, 35–43.

Zarkin, G. A., Dunlap, L. J., & Homsi, G. (2006). The costs of pursuing accreditation for methadone treatment sites. *Evaluation Review, 30*, 119–138.

Zule, W. A., & Desmond, D. P. (1998). Attitudes toward methadone maintenance: Implications for HIV prevention. *Journal of Psychoactive Drugs, 30*(1), 89–97.

Subject Index